A Personal Guide to Living with
Progressive Memory Loss

A Personal Guide to Living with Progressive Memory Loss

Sandy Burgener and Prudence Twigg

Jessica Kingsley Publishers
London and Philadelphia

First published in 2007
by Jessica Kingsley Publishers
116 Pentonville Road
London N1 9JB, UK
and
400 Market Street, Suite 400
Philadelphia, PA 19106, USA

www.jkp.com

Library of Congress Cataloging in Publication Data
Burgener, Sandy, 1947-
  A personal guide to living with progressive memory loss / Sandy Burgener and Prudence Twigg. — 1st American paperback ed.
    p. cm.
  ISBN 978-1-84310-863-4 (pb : alk. paper) 1. Memory disorders—Popular works. 2. Memory disorders in old age—Popular works. I. Twigg, Prudence, 1956- II. Title.
  RC394.M46B87 2008
  616.8'3—dc22
                              2007032761

British Library Cataloguing in Publication Data
A CIP catalogue record for this book is available from the British Library

ISBN 978 1 84310 863 4

Printed and bound in the United States by
Thomson-Shore, Inc.

This book is dedicated to Michelle—one of the finest people we know. After one support group meeting, Michelle, diagnosed with Alzheimer's disease in her late fifties, asked if we had any books she could read to help her learn about her disease. Michelle described how she had been trying to read the books her husband had been reading, but had given up reading them. Michelle did not give up reading the other books because they were too hard for her to understand. She gave up reading them because they were just "too depressing." Michelle, you have always inspired me. Michelle, this book is for you and the many other brave people with memory loss who have touched our lives. May it be uplifting to each of you. As we have said for years in our support groups, you are all truly the bravest people we know.

Acknowledgements

This book is written to honor the hundreds of people with progressive memory loss whom we have met in our clinical practice, research, and support groups over the past 20 years. We are especially grateful to the 96 families that took part in our study of quality of life in memory loss, with some families being in the study for as long as four years. Each person has contributed to our understanding of the needs of these individuals. Each person is represented in this book. We wish we could list each of you by name, as you have each helped shape how we approach the care of people with memory loss. We have become better listeners, clinicians, researchers, advocates, and support group leaders because of our time and conversations with each of you.

We want to acknowledge the support and love of our family and friends, especially our children and husbands. We could not undertake such an important project without the support of the people closest to us. Thank you for your patience, love, and encouragement.

Contents

Introduction

This book has been written for people diagnosed with diseases that cause progressive memory loss and difficulty with thinking. Progressive memory loss can be caused by a number of different changes in the brain, such as those common in Alzheimer's disease, Lewy Body disease, frontal-temporal lobe dementia, or vascular dementia. Alzheimer's disease is the most common cause of progressive memory loss. Despite the growing numbers of people diagnosed with these illnesses, few resources have been developed to aid you in your adjustment to the diagnosis and in managing the disease. This book is intended to begin to fill this gap in resources for you and others affected by progressive memory loss.

No matter what the cause of memory loss and thinking problems, anyone with memory loss will face common issues and concerns as they learn to manage their disease. This book will be most helpful to you in the early stages of your disease, soon after the diagnosis has been made. One goal of this book is to give you a personal resource and guide to help you manage your disease. As common challenges are described, actions you can take to manage the challenge are also given. Not every person will face each issue or challenge described in the book, at least not all at one time. The book can be used at different times throughout the early stages of memory loss, as new or different issues arise. All of the recommendations in the book are based on research findings from studies of people with progressive memory loss. Experiences from the clinical practice of both authors have informed the book as well. The clinical examples are true stories from the authors' practice with older adults with progressive memory loss. So, as you read the book, you will know that the recommendations are based on knowledge—not opinion.

With progressive memory loss, some changes in reading ability may occur. You or your family may think that this means you will not enjoy or benefit from reading. This is not the case. You may have trouble understanding abstract terms and concepts, but you should be able to understand concrete terms and ideas. To help with understanding, we have used examples or illustrations throughout this book. We have also used shorter sentences to convey the main ideas and messages. If an idea or suggestion is complex, we have stated it in several ways to make understanding easier for you. To make sure the book was easily understood, people with memory loss and their family members reviewed chapters as they were written. Their comments and suggestions have been incorporated in the book.

With any disease that is progressive in nature, you may tend to give up or say, "What's the use of trying?" after you receive your diagnosis. Importantly, many treatments, in addition to medications, have been tested and found to be helpful. These treatments may have positive effects on your mental, physical, and emotional functioning. Often, however, these treatments are not discussed with you by your healthcare provider. Recommending medications as the only treatment deprives you of the possible benefits of combining medications with non-medication therapies. We have described many non-medication treatments in this book. By giving you some choices about your treatments, you may have a greater feeling of control over your disease. You can choose which treatments and activities are best for you, in addition to medications. A second goal of this book, then, is to give you and your family members some choices about treatments. Using some of the suggested treatments may help you maintain your thinking abilities and memory longer. So, in addition to being a resource and guide for you, many of the suggested treatments and activities may help you function at the highest level possible as you manage your disease.

While this book is written for people with progressive memory loss, your spouse, family members, and friends might also benefit from reading it. Anyone who knows you well and interacts with you often can gain an understanding of the challenges you are facing. Your family and friends may gain insight into the many possible effects of the diagnosis on you. They will also learn about positive treatments, other than medications, which is especially important for family members and friends to understand. Each person in your life who reads the book may gain a better understanding of how to be a positive support for you. The book can also serve as a basis for talking about your concerns or needs. You may use examples from the book to help describe to others how you feel. As the people around you gain insight into the effects of the disease, they will become better advocates for you and provide stronger support. We are hopeful the book will also benefit you through the insights others will gain about progressive memory loss.

CHAPTER 1

What Progressive Memory Loss Means to You: Claiming the Diagnosis

How do you accept a diagnosis of Alzheimer's disease or any progressive disease that causes loss of memory and interferes with mental functioning? This is a hard question to ask and a harder question to answer. Any progressive disease that affects the ability to think or remember is not easy to face. People receive this diagnosis in a lot of different ways. Some people have said they've felt as though they were "punched in the stomach." Others say the diagnosis is something they never wanted to hear again. Yet, going through the diagnostic process and receiving and accepting a correct diagnosis is the first important step to managing the disease. This chapter describes the process of diagnosing progressive memory loss. Responses to the diagnosis are described, including steps to take after a diagnosis is made.

Why is it important to obtain an accurate diagnosis? First, progressive memory loss can be caused by physical problems that can be treated. Treatable causes of memory loss are often called "reversible" forms of dementia. These treatable physical problems produce symptoms that look like Alzheimer's disease or other causes of progressive memory loss. A very good reason, then, to get an accurate diagnosis is to find and treat other causes of memory loss. Also, an accurate diagnosis helps you to understand the symptoms that you experience on a day-to-day basis. Some people have said that they were almost relieved to know why they had symptoms, including memory loss. Symptoms of progressive memory loss can be vague and difficult to describe. Giving a name to those symptoms can be a relief to the person who is having them.

Another reason to obtain an accurate diagnosis is to receive appropriate treatment. Two types of medications are now approved to treat progressive memory loss, with many more medications being tested. These medications can be especially helpful in the early disease stages. By having an accurate diagnosis, you can seek appropriate medical care to help you manage your everyday symptoms. Many non-medication treatments are also available. You may be able to function better if you receive these combined therapies: medication and non-medication therapy.

Getting an accurate diagnosis helps you plan for your future. It is difficult to plan for your future if you do not know the changes that may lie ahead. Receiving an accurate diagnosis gives you the chance to enroll in a research study testing a new medication or treatment. Many promising treatments for dementia or progressive memory loss take years to study before they receive approval by the Food and Drug Administration (FDA). Enrolling in a research study can give you access to those treatments long before they are available to the general public. A diagnosis of dementia or progressive memory loss will certainly *not* be what you want to hear. However, getting an accurate diagnosis can be helpful to you and your family.

Getting a diagnosis

How does a person go about obtaining an accurate diagnosis? First of all, an accurate diagnosis requires a very thorough history and physical examination. This examination includes an evaluation of your physical health, including a screening for any physical cause for the changes in your memory and mental ability. The examination will also include a very thorough testing of your mental ability. This testing assesses any impairment you might have in your short-term or long-term memory, judgment, perceptions, and reasoning. The healthcare provider will also conduct blood tests to look for physical problems that may be causing your symptoms. The blood tests will screen for things such as anemia, abnormal blood chemical levels, or high or low blood sugar levels. Generally, the healthcare provider will also order a brain scan, which will be either in the form of a computer-assisted tomography (CAT) scan or magnetic resonance imaging (MRI). These basic tests are commonly done to make a correct diagnosis. As you can see, this testing requires more than the usual 15–20 minute office visit! Approved testing centers are available across the USA and in other countries. These approved centers provide a standard diagnostic evaluation that meets well-accepted guidelines for the assessment. Additional psychological tests may be given in these national testing centers to identify exactly what disorder is causing the mental and memory symptoms. More intensive examinations, such as a spinal tap or positron emission tomography (PET) scan, may also be given. These additional tests take more time, but help to assure us that the correct diagnosis has been reached.

Just as physical disorders can cause changes in mental ability and memory, medications taken to treat other illnesses can actually cause these symptoms. The diagnostic evaluation should include a review of medications you are currently taking. Often, changing or stopping a medication can reduce your symptoms. This change can occur without increasing your risk of a decline in your physical health. A thorough diagnostic evaluation results in a correct diagnosis about 90 percent of the time. New tests are now available that will increase the accuracy of the diagnoses to even more than 90 percent.

You and your spouse or supportive family member may need to be assertive to assure you receive a thorough and appropriate diagnostic evaluation. It is not uncommon for healthcare providers to dismiss symptoms of progressive memory loss as just "normal aging." Often, you and your family members may know that what you are experiencing is not "normal," but is more problematic. One wife of a member of my support group for people with early-stage memory loss recounted her frustration at obtaining a correct diagnosis for her husband, Ray. Ray's internist was not "tuned in" to dementia or other causes of memory loss. Each time Ray visited the internist, he would give Ray the basic10-item Mini-Mental State Examination (MMSE), which Ray completed accurately. The doctor then felt he had no need for a further evaluation or for treatment for Ray's symptoms. This delay in receiving an accurate diagnosis resulted in a delay in starting the right medications for Ray's disease. Although we want to trust that every healthcare provider understands memory loss, this may not be the case. Assertive action and questioning by you and your family may be necessary to assure a complete assessment and an accurate diagnosis is reached.

Responses to the diagnosis

The process of obtaining an accurate diagnosis for the cause of progressive memory loss can actually be positive for the person. Well-trained and sensitive healthcare providers can help you feel at ease during the evaluation. You may even find the evaluation interesting. In some cases, however, the evaluation can be a less positive experience. Knowing what to expect, however, can prepare you for some possible negative emotions and responses. For example, some terms used during the diagnostic evaluation may be difficult for you to hear. Terms such as "victim," "sufferer," or "demented" are dehumanizing. Hearing these terms may cause you to have a negative emotional response. These terms also place you in a position where you feel as if you are being put upon rather than having any control over what is happening to you. Sadly, these terms are still used both in the diagnostic evaluation and in written information about the disease. If you feel the diagnostic process was difficult or impersonal, you are not alone. Studies have shown that very few people are satisfied with their diagnostic evaluation. Some people have described it as being overly negative. Some physicians don't discuss what can be done to treat something like dementia or progressive memory loss. Instead, the disease is viewed as a condition of old age. When medications are prescribed, healthcare providers may fail to fully describe the side effects and benefits of the drugs. Understanding how the drugs work and possible benefits is important as many people get discouraged when they have side effects. If you do not know how to manage side effects or understand the benefits of the medications, you may decide to stop taking medications that can provide positive results.

Often, during the diagnostic evaluation healthcare providers might address their questions or explanations to a family member rather than to you. The lack of opportunity to be heard during the diagnostic testing may increase your frustration. Being devalued in this way may contribute to your negative responses to the experience. Although it is important for healthcare providers to talk to family members, you should be included in the conversation. Your input and responses should be obtained throughout the examination. You should also be informed of what tests are being done and why. This information will help you be more comfortable throughout the evaluation.

A very common response to the diagnosis is one of shock and disbelief. Members of my support group have described responses such as, "It has taken me years to get used to the idea of having this disease" or "I couldn't believe it was true until the doctor said it. I really didn't feel any different than I had before." Some describe their responses in physical terms, such as feeling as if someone "dropped a brick on my head." One woman in my support group described the process as being extremely threatening and dehumanizing. Students were present during the evaluation, although no one asked her per-mission to allow student observers. She felt that this contributed to her feelings of loss of control and powerlessness. She also felt that her privacy was invaded. Another person in my support group said that she received the diagnosis from her physician over the phone—something that should *not* happen in today's healthcare system. Negative responses to the diagnostic evaluation often can-not be prevented. The benefits from receiving an accurate diagnosis, however, should outweigh the negative parts of the evaluation.

Ideally, the diagnostic evaluation will be conducted by a highly skilled and knowledgeable healthcare provider. Often, this provider is a specialist such as a neurologist or geriatric specialist. Physicians in other specialties may have the knowledge and experience needed to carry out a thorough evaluation. Other healthcare providers, such as advanced practice nurses and physician's assis-tants, may also be highly skilled in the diagnostic process. Generally, health providers from different fields work as a team to assure a thorough and accurate diagnostic evaluation. For example, a psychologist may conduct a screening for depression while a neurologist may do the assessment of mental functioning and memory. In the ideal diagnostic evaluation, you will have time to ask ques-tions at every step in the process. While a highly skilled healthcare provider is important, it is also essential that the diagnosis be carried out in a humane and non-threatening manner. Approved diagnostic centers use professionals from different specialties to carry out the diagnostic evaluation. You may learn about these centers by contacting your local Alzheimer's Association in the USA or the Alzheimer's Society in Canada and specialty groups in other countries.

Following the diagnostic evaluation, the findings are often shared in a family conference. It is helpful for you and your family members to hear the same information and have the opportunity to ask questions. During this conference, the healthcare provider may talk with you about what to expect in your future. Also, treatment options should be carefully explained especially the medication and non-medication treatments that are available. Opportunities to participate in research studies may also be offered to you at this time. Support services may be described. These services can include things such as support groups or education, and therapies such as cognitive or behavioral therapy. Participating in wellness programs such as exercise, creative activities, and social events can also provide positive benefits. These wellness programs are described in a later chapter in this book. Generally, openness and honesty about your treatment choices leads to the best outcomes for you and your family.

As the person most affected by the diagnosis, it is your right to be involved in your care and decision-making, as long as you are able. Understanding what the disease means and what to expect in the future allows you to speak for yourself. Knowing what to expect allows you to make more informed decisions about what you want to do today and in your future. You may also take positive actions to protect your own quality of life. In addition to giving you the information you need to plan for your future, other positive responses to the diagnosis have been expressed. Some people are relieved to finally understand their symptoms and say things such as, "Now I understand why I felt the way I did." Others have been grateful to know that they are not "contagious" and that their symptoms will not transfer to their family members. Understanding the disease and its effects on you can provide you with knowledge and insight into your symptoms, allowing you to move on to the next step in managing the disease.

The acceptance of the diagnosis for some is not totally negative. Some people with progressive memory loss talk a good deal about past positive times. Others find reassurance in the close relationships and love they receive from important people in their lives. Some learn to accept the loss of abilities inherent in memory loss. Instead of asking "Why me?" some cherish the good parts of their lives both in the present and in the past. Often, it is easy to focus on the negative when receiving such a life-changing diagnosis. A totally negative view, however, may prevent you from enjoying and valuing the positive parts of your life that are ahead.

What next: informing others of the diagnosis

Early in most diseases that cause progressive memory loss, individuals with the diagnosis can function and perform much as they have in the past. As outward appearance is not changed, the person can carry on much as they have in the past, especially during brief encounters. In fact, many individuals describe how they cover up their symptoms. People with memory loss often fear rejection or undue sympathy from others if the diagnosis is revealed. Those in my support group have described some fairly elaborate strategies they developed to succeed in social situations. These cover-up strategies prevent them from telling others of the diagnosis—at least for a while. However, the energy and concentration required to cover up symptoms will eventually become tiring. In fact, some people will stop going out socially owing to their fear that they will no longer be able to carry out their cover up with success. Covering or hiding your symptoms may be successful for a short time. However, the long-term result may be less energy and eventual withdrawal from interactions with others. Being open and honest with others about the diagnosis is a positive alternative that you may want to consider to prevent negative outcomes.

Positive results can come from giving your spouse or other family members permission to share your diagnosis with others. You may set limits on whom you are willing to share the diagnosis with. Being open and honest about your wishes may make it easier for family members to ensure your needs are met while allowing them to maintain social relationships with others. By sharing the diagnosis with trusted friends and family members, you will allow your family members more freedom while you surround yourself with caring people.

Stories of sharing the diagnosis

Below are the stories of two people who were diagnosed with Alzheimer's disease. Both were healthy and active men in their early seventies. One, Dale, decided to share his diagnosis with family members and friends, with positive results. The second man, Robert, kept his diagnosis a secret for a long as possible, with less positive results.

Dale's story

Dale was a retired professor of theology who had taught at a local seminary for most of his career. He was well known and loved by the community, including a large group of former students and active pastors. Although Dale had held a prestigious position throughout most of his life, he decided to be open about his diagnosis of Alzheimer's disease. His wife assisted him in writing a letter to his trusted colleagues, friends, and family members. In some cases, Dale and his wife went to dinner or invited friends to their home to share the diagnosis. Throughout this time, Dale was constantly pleased by the understanding he received from those who learned of his diagnosis. Dale experienced a sense of prayerful support from those around him. This support and understanding allowed Dale to remain socially active without fear of embarrassment or a need to cover up his symptoms. This support provided Dale and his wife comfort and pleasure through the years after his diagnosis.

George's story

George lived in a small farming community where he had raised his family and lived most of his life. George was active in a number of different community groups and held some leadership roles in his church. He was a very social person, and enjoyed dancing and sharing his humor with others. Because George lived in a small town, he was also fearful of news or gossip spreading about his diagnosis of Alzheimer's disease. He said the news would "spread like wildfire" and possibly cause him embarrassment. George and his wife attended the support group I led in a city about 40 miles away from George's hometown. During the first few years George attended the group, he talked a great deal about his concern over sharing his diagnosis. He also talked about the anxiety he had when he went out. George would describe the extreme measures he took to cover up his symptoms. He sadly refused to go to many social events for fear he would say or do something suspicious. In the end, not telling others about his diagnosis caused George to have a great deal of unnecessary worry and to withdraw. As George was an exceptionally social and outgoing person, hiding his diagnosis and staying home lessened his quality of life at a time when he very much enjoyed the companionship of others.

In a book, *My Journey into Alzheimer's Disease* (Davis and Davis, 1989), Robert Davis describes his reactions to the responses of those around him following his diagnosis:

> As soon as my diagnosis was announced, some people became uncomfortable around me. I realized that the shock and pain are difficult to deal with at first. It was strange that in most cases, I had to make the effort to seek out people who were avoiding me and look them in the eye and say, 'I

> don't bite. I'm still the same person. I just can't do my work any more. I
> know that one of these days I will not be here any more, but for now I am
> still home, and here, and I need your friendship and acceptance. (p.100)

People with progressive memory loss often do not anticipate these reactions from long-time friends and co-workers. Understanding why these reactions occur can help to ease your disappointment when they do happen.

The responses of others to the disease diagnosis, such as those described above, often raise concerns about whom to tell and when to tell others. No set rules or guidelines exist for exactly whom you should tell about your diagnosis. The decision regarding whom to tell is often made with both the individual with progressive memory loss and close family members. Generally, your closest friends and relatives will benefit from knowing about the diagnosis. Without understanding your symptoms, friends and family members may become uncomfortable around you. They may have difficulty understanding the changes, however slight, they see in you. Even with the best plan regarding whom to tell, some people will respond negatively to you when told about your diagnosis. These negative responses may be attributed to a number of different factors. Some people fear that they may be diagnosed with such a disorder themselves—so your diagnosis is "too close for comfort." Others may not understand progressive memory loss and may be unsure how to approach you. Generally, people who have been supportive in the past will be very understanding of the diagnosis. Most people will be grateful that you have trusted them and have shared the diagnosis with them. Some will be relieved, as they will understand the subtle changes they may have seen in you. Overall, most people will be accepting and willing to help in any way possible. Telling others and accepting the diagnosis yourself allows you to benefit from the help of others. Learning to accept these positive acts of kindness provides a good starting point for continuing to accept help from those who care about you.

Just as there are no set rules about when to tell others, no definite guidelines exist about how to tell others about the diagnosis. You will probably choose whatever method is most comfortable for you. You may decide that a face-to-face talk with close friends and relatives is best. Your most trusted and valued friends and relatives may be the first you will choose to tell. These will be the people with whom you will be most comfortable and relaxed. They might also be the people who will respond in a positive and supportive way. Or, you might decide that sending a letter to those close to you is more comfortable. You may want to use your Christmas card list as one way of identifying those people in your life who are important and who would want to know. Both methods have advantages and disadvantages. In a face-to-face talk, others have the chance to ask questions directly of you. They also have the opportunity to talk with you about how they might be helpful. Using a letter, everyone learns of the diagnosis at the same time. Learning the truth at the same time may prevent undue gossip or incorrect information being passed from one person to another. Using either a conversation or letter, in *Alzheimer's Early Stages: First Steps for Family, Friends and Caregivers,* Daniel Kuhn (2003) suggests that the following information be shared with others.

1. Medical facts about the disease and diagnosis.

2. Symptoms that you might be experiencing, such as memory loss.

3. Needs that you have, such as assistance with transportation.

4. Examples of how others might be helpful.

5. The importance of staying involved in your life.

6. Continuing to be caring.

You will want to personalize the letter, of course. You may want to describe how important it is to you to continue your relationships with others. You may also want to describe the types of social interactions that are most comfortable to you, such as dining out in small groups, going to movies, and so on. Many of your friends and family members will want to be helpful. If you give them suggestions, they will often be pleased that they can assist in some way.

Any traumatic event, such as a diagnosis of progressive memory loss, can alter relationships. In some cases, the new challenges in a relationship can bring out the best in people. You may find that you are actually closer to some relatives and friends than you were before your diagnosis. You—and others—may value the time together more and find pleasure in life's everyday occurrences. An older woman in my support group often described the changes in her relationship with her grandchildren, saying, "Sure, they know that I'm not quite like I was before. Sometimes, I can tell—they look at me and are trying to figure out what I'm saying. But we have fun. We laugh a lot. We enjoy our time together more than we ever did before." Another person, a retired physician, described the pleasure he found in fishing with his son: "We used to spend time together with the family, but that wasn't the same. Now my son comes to see me every week. We fish together most of the day. Sometimes we talk. Sometimes we just fish. But we both enjoy being together. I haven't felt this close to my son for many years."

Many family members or friends may find strengths in their relationship with you that were not there before. Being open and honest about the diagnosis allows for these positive outcomes as well as the negative ones. You will learn quickly not to spend time being concerned about those people who drift away or are uncomfortable with you. Your time and energy will be much better spent if you focus on those with whom you find joy and comfort.

Interventions to assist with acceptance of the diagnosis
Support groups

Support groups for people with progressive memory loss are becoming more available. These groups serve those with the diagnosis, rather than family members. The groups are designed to provide emotional and psychological support, education, and a place to share common concerns. Groups generally consist of 10–15 individuals with memory loss and professional leaders. Confidentiality is expected so that participants can feel free to share information and experiences openly and honestly. The frequency with which the group meets varies, generally from once a week to twice a month. Participation in a support group is especially helpful after the diagnosis. This is the time when you have many questions and are attempting to adapt to the challenges inherent in any chronic illness.

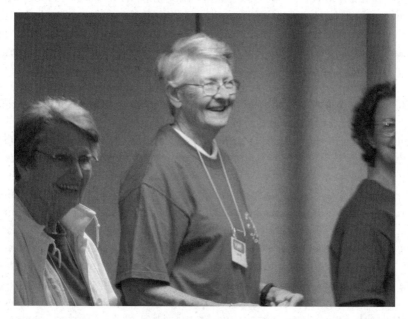

People attending support groups tend to identify quickly with the other group members. As they all share common issues and concerns, the group members' discussions can be very helpful. You may also have a sense of a "shared experience." A diagnosis of progressive memory loss can tend to separate you from others through your own actions or the withdrawal of others. The support and shared experiences inherent in the support group provides you with a sense of not being alone. Group members tend to be very empathetic with one another, having faced similar or like concerns. They are also excellent resources. Each person manages their symptoms and challenges in different ways. Therefore, the collective wisdom of the group can provide helpful guidance. Members of my support group have noted, "This is the one place where I feel free to say what I think" or "We all care about each other here—I know I will be accepted here." One group member's wife related to me that her husband did not always know the day of the week. However, he did know which day was the day for his support group meeting. The group had become such a part of his life that he instinctively knew the day the meeting would be held. Even with memory loss, group members will ask about one another if someone is missing—the members come to mean so much to one another. Often, other groups will form with members of the support group. For example, group members have begun to meet for meals around special holidays or events. This extension of the group allows for added support while providing fun activities that are comfortable. Being part of a support group is an excellent way to help you as you accept your diagnosis of progressive memory loss.

Friendship and social groups

One mistake many people make when diagnosed with progressive memory loss is to give up too much, too soon. As described before, you may find yourself wanting to withdraw from groups or social events for fear that you will embarrass yourself. You may also fear being hurt by someone's negative comments. Withdrawing may seem to be a safe way of managing your symptoms and protecting your self-esteem. Also, most adults want to maintain their independence—at any cost. If you are unable to drive, you may choose to stay home rather than ask someone to give you a ride. One the other hand, you have probably been a part of some groups or activities that have meant a lot to you. These groups may be card clubs, choir or church-related groups, or service organizations such as Elks, Rotary, or the Woman's Club. The people that make up these groups and other close friends may be a big part of your social circle. Giving up these friendships and activities may appear to be the easiest path. However, the long-term effects of withdrawing from friends and social groups may leave you feeling lonely, sad, and even depressed.

Research has shown that the more a person with progressive memory loss stays involved in past activities, the better are the long-term outcomes. While some friends may disappoint or hurt you, other friends will continue to be sources of comfort and companionship. An older man, retired from years of working on the railroad in a small, rural town, said, "With this disease, you find out who your true friends are! And, that's not so bad." You cannot prevent friends from withdrawing. You can, however, enjoy and continue to be part of groups that understand and welcome you. Your true friends will find ways to be with you that are enjoyable for you both. For example, a single woman in our support group took vacations with a lifelong friend each year—traveling around 600 miles to the east coast. When she felt like the trip was too difficult, her friend found vacation spots that were much closer to home. In this way, the dear friends were able to continue their yearly vacations. Friends and close family members will want to continue to be part of your life. Many will find ways to make it possible for you to continue doing the things you love.

At various times, I have asked the members of our support group what they would like most to tell their friends and family members about themselves. The most common response is, "I want to be treated as I have always been treated. I am the same person that I was before the diagnosis. I haven't changed who I am, so please don't treat me as if I'm different." If you feel the same way, you may want to share this with your friends and family members. Knowing how you feel allows them to feel more comfortable, making your time together more positive. Being open and honest with the important people in your life allows you to stay involved with the people and activities that mean the most.

Treating depression

Despite your best efforts, you may find yourself feeling sad or depressed about your diagnosis. In fact, depression is generally more of a concern. You may feel at first that you should handle your sadness yourself—that your feelings are in your control. However, if you notice that your sadness affects how you live your everyday life, then you might want to seek professional help. Extreme sadness or depression can affect many parts of your everyday functioning, such as your sleep, appetite, energy level, willingness to be with others, or ability to think clearly and make decisions. You may also believe that these symptoms are part of the diagnosis of progressive memory loss. In fact, you can have a depression *in addition* to progressive memory loss. However, if the depression is treated, your symptoms will be lessened. Fewer symptoms allow you to function better.

Some people with progressive memory loss think that being sad or depressed goes along with their disease. Although about 50 percent of those with memory loss will have some depression, depression is *not* considered to be a normal part of the condition. The depression should be treated. Your physician or primary healthcare provider may be the place to start. Your physician may elect to treat you or to refer you to a specialist, usually a psychologist or psychiatrist. Several treatment options are available. A combined therapy might include both medications and individual or group counseling. Successful treatment will result in an improved mood. The symptoms that go along with depression should also be relieved. Even though you still may feel sad at times, the sadness you will feel will not be as severe as depression. The normal sadness that goes along with adjusting to any chronic illness will also not affect your functioning as much as depression. Treating depression allows you to manage your everyday life more positively, increasing your quality of life.

Planning for the future: threat or challenge?

For many people, the diagnosis of progressive memory loss comes at a time in their life when they had planned for a rewarding and happy retirement. You may have planned to do those things you had always wanted to do and never had time for before. Then, suddenly, a diagnosis you could never imagine happens to you. This diagnosis is often what people think of as happening to "someone else—not me." This disruption to your plans can cause anger, frustration, and resentment. When this negative response occurs, the diagnosis is viewed as a threat.

An alternative response is to view the diagnosis as a challenge. Seeing the challenges in the diagnosis allows you to respond in an entirely different way. Instead of being angry and discouraged, you will find yourself problem-solving and planning for your future in a different way. The diagnosis of progressive memory loss does not mean that your future plans cannot be fulfilled. The diagnosis more often means that you will need to do some things differently, adapting your activities to your abilities. Viewing the diagnosis as a challenge allows you to proceed with life in a more positive, productive way.

Research on coping with stress tells us that most people will respond in one of these two ways to a stressful event. People will either see the stressful event as a threat or challenge. Certainly, receiving a diagnosis of progressive memory loss is stressful. Receiving the diagnosis is also something you have no control over. How you respond to that stress is in your control, however. You can decide to view the diagnosis as either a threat or challenge. Viewing the diagnosis as a challenge allows you to go on with your life in a much more positive way than if you choose to view the diagnosis as a threat. Viewing the diagnosis as a challenge does not mean, of course, that you will have an easy path to follow. The word "challenge" itself suggests obstacles and hard choices. "Challenge" also suggests responses characterized by strength, determination, and wisdom. I have often told the people in our support group that they are the bravest people I know. The journey of progressive memory loss or dementia may not be easy. However, the journey may be rewarding at times. The journey can also be filled with the people and activities you love and value the most.

CHAPTER 2

Maintaining Personhood

A diagnosis of irreversible memory loss or dementia can affect how a person views themselves—often defined as one's sense of "personhood." The changes that go along with a diagnosis of progressive memory loss can directly affect how you feel about yourself. These changes can make you feel uncertain about your future. This uncertainty makes it hard to imagine what you will be like in the future—affecting your sense of personhood. You may find yourself asking, "Who am I now?" and "Who will I be in the future?" Thomas Kitwood (1997a, 1997b), a pioneer in the care of people with progressive memory loss, was one of the first people to help us understand why maintaining a sense of personhood is so important. When personhood is maintained, you may continue to have a high quality of life, even with changing abilities and uncertainty. Kitwood views personhood as much more than the ability to remember. In other words, each one of us is defined by much more than our thinking or reasoning ability. Kitwood defines personhood as being the "status bestowed upon one human being by others" (p.18). In this definition, personhood is defined by our relationships, our social being, and our ability to feel for and respond to others. Personhood implies recognition from others, respect, and mutual trust. Using this definition, it is easy to see how personhood can be maintained, even with a disease that can impair memory or thinking ability. Your ability to relate to others and to respond to others in loving and caring ways can remain a part of who you are as a person.

Other individuals with progressive memory loss or dementia have written about how they experience threats to their personhood. In her book, *Living in the Labyrinth: A Personal Journey through the Maze of Alzheimer's* (1993), Dianne McGowin describes her own struggle to maintain her personhood. Dianne also describes her desire to hold on to a sense of herself and her dignity, despite the disease diagnosis. She says:

> If I am no longer a woman, why do I still feel like one? If I am no longer worth holding, why do I crave it? If I am no longer sensual, why do I enjoy the soft texture of silk against my skin? If I am no longer sensitive, why do moving song lyrics strike a responsive chord in me? My every molecule

seems to scream out that I do, indeed, exist and that existence must be valued by someone. (McGowin, 1993, p.123–4)

Dianne describes her awareness of the need to keep a sense of personhood, including the sensual and feminine aspects of herself. This awareness can assist those with memory loss to keep a sense of personhood, as they stay in touch with their feelings, desires, and values.

Cary Henderson (1998), author of *Partial View: An Alzheimer's Journey*, describes his response to the effects of the disease on his personhood. Professor Henderson states:

> It's a very come and go disease. When I make a blunder, I tend to get defensive about it. I have a sense of shame for not knowing what I should have known. And, for not being able to think things and see things that I saw several years ago, when I was a "normal" person. But everybody, by this time, knows that I'm not a normal person. And, I'm quite aware of that. (p.36)

This account of the experience of progressive memory loss hints at the effect of the disease on one's sense of personhood. "Normal" may be a comparison of oneself to others. "Normal" may also be a comparison of oneself in the present to oneself prior to the diagnosis. This need for normalcy is strong. What is normal for any person can assist in defining their continuing personhood. Although certain skills and abilities may change with the disease, the need for normalcy and an enduring sense of personhood remains strong.

This chapter focuses on how your sense of self or personhood can be affected by your diagnosis. Some interventions will be described to give you ways to help maintain your sense of self. As your self-esteem can be affected by a loss of self and negative aspects of progressive memory loss, we describe ways to maintain your self-esteem. The purpose of this chapter is to provide you with different approaches to minimize the effects of the disease on your view of self. By assisting you to maintain a positive sense of personhood, a higher quality of life is possible.

How personhood is affected by progressive memory loss

Personhood can be influenced by a number of changes that go along with a diagnosis of progressive memory loss. Changes often occur in the social environment in which you interact. How others respond to you as a person with memory loss can have a powerful effect on your sense of personhood and self-esteem. As you interact with others, if they tend to be uncomfortable or focus on losses, it will be more difficult for you to feel positive about yourself. Friends and previous acquaintances will often "drop off" or decrease their contacts with you—regardless of your efforts. These negative interactions and loss of previous friendships make it difficult to focus on the positive aspects of yourself and the strengths that you retain. In this way, the social environment is a powerful force in how you maintain your sense of personhood. The degree to which you are able to stay positive about yourself, to some extent, is dictated by the healthy response of others. In this sense, your personhood is not so much affected by the disease as by the social situations in which you find yourself and the responses of those with whom you interact.

A second aspect of progressive memory loss that affects personhood is a loss of abilities. One effect of progressive memory loss or dementia is a loss of ability to do some tasks and previous role functions. For example, you may have always been the person in your family to manage the finances, schedule activities, or drive when traveling. The effects of the disease on the brain may cause you to lose some ability to carry out tasks of this type. So often, members of my support group will describe how these losses impact their self-esteem and personhood. One member continually describes himself as feeling useless as he is no longer able to drive his wife as he had done for many years. Another gentleman in the group often states he is just "not the man he once was" as he can no longer work in the job he held for many years. A very successful teacher, Carol, often said, "I *used* to be Phi Beta Kappa." Of course, the diagnosis of progressive memory loss did not take away Carol's status as being Phi Beta Kappa—she just felt that she could no longer claim this part of herself. A loss of ability can cause you to change how you view yourself as a person. Also, loss of ability can cause you to feel more dependent on others—a feeling most of us resist during most of our adolescent and adult lives. Later in this chapter some strategies to lessen the effects of loss on your sense of self will be described.

A third effect of the disease diagnosis on personhood is loss of control. Changes in your social status and abilities are often out of your direct control. You may then begin to sense an overall loss of control over your life. This loss of control can be both frustrating and demoralizing for you. As adults, we like to have control over our daily lives, including our schedules, routines, and activities. With progressive memory loss, well-meaning spouses and family members may assume responsibility for tasks you were used to doing—a reversal of how you are accustomed to functioning! While you may want and need assistance at times, you may also find yourself resenting someone else doing something you enjoyed and have done for most of your adult life. Most of all, you will probably want things to be normal—to have control over how your life functions. No longer being able to control events in your daily life may leave you with a general sense of loss of personhood and a need to redefine normalcy.

Benefits of maintained personhood

When personhood is maintained with progressive memory loss, a number of positive outcomes are possible. As you continue to be a social person and relate to others, you may continue to be included in the everyday lives of those around you. Your presence will be valued and desired. With maintained personhood, the parts of yourself that are unique—that define you as "one of a kind"—will also most likely be retained. We know from research that people with progressive memory loss are most likely to hold on to the skills and knowledge that they used most in their life. These skills and knowledge are different for each person, and help to define how each individual differs from the next. Keeping a positive sense of personhood also helps you to withstand the effects of the disease on your everyday functioning. If you know who you are in relation to others and have a positive view of yourself, you are more likely to adapt to these changes in a positive way. In other words, maintained personhood means more than just being happier. Maintaining your personhood can help you manage the effects of your disease in a positive way—leading to improved quality of life for both you and those you love.

In this chapter some actions or interventions will be described to help you preserve your sense of personhood. First, a true story of retained personhood will be described, followed by a true story of a situation where the sense of personhood was lost. The stories include examples of ways to maintain personhood.

John's story

One positive example of retained personhood comes from a retired veteran who has participated in my support group for several years. During this time, this independent gentleman, John, has maintained involvement in many of the retired-military activities he enjoyed prior to his diagnosis. Even after he lost his ability to drive, John learned to use the public transportation system to attend meetings and other veteran-related activities. When it came time to move into an assisted living facility, John was active in visiting the different facilities. By visiting each facility himself, John was able to let his children know his preferences—based on first-hand knowledge. From his residence, John continued to remain active in veteran affairs through his writing of letters to legislators and to the editor of the local newspaper. He also continued to participate in church-related activities, allowing him the religious support and expression he had enjoyed throughout his life. John would travel by bus to visit his children and grandchildren who lived too far away for regular visiting. By keeping involved and active in previous roles, John was able to maintain his sense of himself—as a veteran, as a church member, as leader of his family, and as an active member of the community. Staying engaged also allowed John to maintain his sense of control over his life and the normalcy he desired.

Several things can be learned from this story. By using many of the interventions described later in this chapter, John was able to keep a sense of who he was as a person. John was active and took some responsibility for his own welfare. He was able to look at what he valued most about his life and he then designed ways to keep those parts of his life active and alive. John's actions helped him maintain his personhood, even when he lost some of his abilities, such as driving and short-term memory. John was able to maintain a positive outlook as he was able to keep his sense of personhood.

Ruth's story

An example of loss of personhood comes from a person who was also once very independent and self-sufficient. Ruth was a widow who continued to live in the small town where she and her husband had raised their children and later retired. Soon after her diagnosis of Alzheimer's disease, Ruth's children decided they wanted her to live with them. Ruth gave in to their suggestions, although she really wanted to live in the small town where she and her husband had raised their family, where she was involved in church, and where most of her friends lived. Although both her children wanted to spend time with Ruth, they were employed and had little room in their homes for another person. So, the solution was to have Ruth spend three months with one child and then three months with the other—alternating between the two homes. With this arrangement, Ruth was unable to continue in any of the activities she once enjoyed. She soon lost contact with old friends. By going from one home to the other, Ruth was not able to establish a space she could call her own. Also, as Ruth lost her ability to care for herself, she began to feel as if she was a burden to both children. This feeling of being a burden eventually affected Ruth's self-esteem. Ruth experienced a sense of total loss of control over her life. She also lost her sense of what was normal for her, as her new lifestyle was very different from how she had functioned in the past. Even when Ruth could function very well, she became discouraged about her situation, often referring to herself as a burden and longing for the life she had known.

In this example, Ruth's personhood was negatively affected by loss of contact with previously positive people in her life. The lack of opportunity for Ruth to engage in previous activities contributed to her loss of personhood. Constantly moving between the homes of her two children prevented Ruth from establishing herself in new relationships. She was not able to establish a daily routine that fit her past schedule, as she was always trying to fit into her children's schedules. Loss of abilities contributed to Ruth's feelings of loss of control as well. Without contact with past friends, positive interactions, and control over her living situation, Ruth was unable to maintain a positive view of herself. All of these factors contributed to Ruth's loss of personhood.

Interventions to maintain personhood

As described in John's story, it is possible to maintain a positive sense of self and personhood—even in the face of progressive memory loss or dementia. Several interventions and self-care actions will be described to assist you to maintain your sense of self. These interventions will also assist you in keeping a positive view of yourself and to focus on your abilities.

Managing negative thoughts and responses

One way to help maintain self-esteem is to avoid becoming habitually negative about yourself. Often, when we encounter negative responses from others, we tend to respond negatively ourselves. This negative emotional response can eventually result in distorted thinking—or an overly negative view of ourselves. For example, someone in your family may have asked you to pick up something on your way home from a meeting or to stop and get something for them while you were out. You may have totally forgotten to commit this to memory and because your memory is not as good as before it may have more easily slipped your mind. So you might get home and the person might say to you, "Well, do you have what I asked you to get?" So you immediately find yourself feeling stupid, as if you have let someone down, and you may blame yourself for not being able to remember long enough to "do it right." This sense of not being able to get it right can result in an overgeneralization of this one very small incident. You may even find yourself saying, "Well, I've just become an incompetent person." So you have gone from forgetting to do a small task to feeling totally incompetent. You might think this example is an exaggeration of how individuals with memory loss really respond. However, this negative response happens often, especially when you are adjusting to the diagnosis and memory loss. Because memory assists you with your actions in so many ways, it is easy to let these little events overtake how you feel about yourself. You may develop a negative view of yourself because of this overgeneralization.

Some simple strategies will help you to keep from allowing these small incidents from making you feel negative about yourself. You can use these strategies whenever you find yourself feeling negative, exaggerating the negative emotions you feel, or thinking that one negative response means you are incompetent. Using these strategies will assist you in maintaining a positive view of yourself, as well as your personhood.

Avoid focusing on the negative

One way to deal with your negative responses is to be more objective when mistakes happen—and they will happen. If you make a small mistake, it is helpful to be as objective as you can about it. Try to think about what happened realistically. Instead of saying to yourself, "I'm really stupid; I forgot this." Say to yourself, "I know I have difficulty with my memory. I was focusing on getting where I wanted to go and back home safely. I was trying to make sure that I didn't forget anybody's name at the meeting. So it was probably not realistic for me to expect myself to remember one more thing." This more realistic response is probably much closer to the truth than your negative feelings. Being more objective about what happened can keep you from thinking that if one thing goes wrong, then everything is negative. More objective thinking will help you not blame yourself or feel overly negative.

Avoid all-or-nothing thinking

Using words such as "should" and "shouldn't" often happens as you interact with other people. Others may tend to blame you or put you in a position where you feel responsible when you do not live up to their expectations. A very real example of this was shared in our support group. One very independent woman in her mid-sixties, Jane, described how her son made her feel in a recent telephone conversation. Jane's son had called her several days before our meeting and had asked her to do a specific task: get a bus pass for an upcoming doctor's visit. The son called a couple days later and asked Jane if she had gotten the bus pass. Jane said, with some guilt, "Oh no, I'm sorry I forgot all about that. No, I didn't follow up on that." Her son's response was, "Well, Mom, I just asked you to do that two days ago. How could you have forgotten?" Jane ended the conversation feeling upset at herself and telling herself she "shouldn't" have forgotten what her son had asked. Jane was placing a "should" on herself—and feeling as if she had failed her son. Jane's son contributed to her negative response without really intending to hurt her.

In discussing this incident in the group, Jane became aware of how she had allowed this one small incident to make her feel negative about herself. She was also dreading the next time she was to talk with her son, fearing she would say something wrong. The group suggested that the next time this happened, Jane could say to her son, "I've been diagnosed with memory loss, so of course I'm going to have trouble remembering. I'm not sure you should expect me to remember something that you told me two days ago." The group talked with Jane about how to avoid making herself feel as if she should do something that was not realistic for her. When you find yourself saying words like "should" or "shouldn't," it may be helpful to ask yourself: "Is this really something I *should* have done, or is it something I can no longer expect of myself?" "Do I expect too much of myself?" "Do my family members and friends expect too much of me as well?" If you answer these questions honestly, you may find yourself using the words "should" and "shouldn't" less often.

Avoid blaming yourself for things you cannot control
One response that happens after a diagnosis of progressive memory loss is the tendency to blame yourself when things do not go well. In the example described above, the support group helped Jane to see that her forgetfulness was not her fault. She could not control the memory loss. Also, if Jane did not think to write a reminder to herself, this may have been caused by something that distracted her at the time. As Jane's memory loss is not her fault, the result of her forgetting is something she should not blame herself for. If you find you blame yourself when you forget or when things go wrong, try to be realistic about what you expect of yourself. If the effects of the disease have contributed to a negative outcome, then the outcome truly is not your fault. Avoiding blaming yourself for things you cannot control will help you keep a positive and more realistic view of yourself. This view will also help you maintain your sense of personhood.

Cognitive-behavioral therapies
Cognitive-behavioral therapies are used often to help maintain personhood with progressive memory loss. Linda Teri and colleagues (Teri and Gallagher-Thompson 1991) have used these therapies since the early 1990s to help manage the negative responses to the disease. Cognitive therapies help people with progressive memory loss to correct exaggerated negative thoughts and replace them with more accurate, positive thinking. Cognitive therapists assist those with memory loss to view negative interactions in a more realistic way. The therapies also give individuals with memory loss coping skills for

dealing with the negative responses of others. The behavioral therapies assist people with memory loss to stay active in positive and pleasant experiences. By focusing on what you have enjoyed in the past, behavioral therapies help you identify what activities are important for you to continue. This combined therapy then assists with maintaining personhood by helping you stay active and involved with positive activities, while decreasing your negative feelings about yourself.

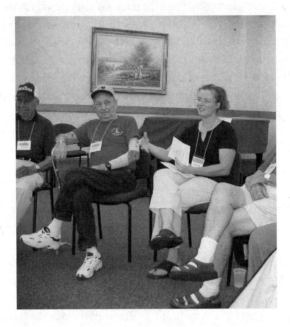

Cognitive-behavioral therapies are also useful for identifying your strengths and abilities. For example, many people with memory loss feel guilty if they use lists or cues as reminders of things to do or events that they are likely to forget. Cognitive-behavioral therapies help you see that using lists or cues is nothing to feel guilty about, but is a positive way to function at the highest level possible. Suggestions or strategies are often offered to help you avoid situations that may be negative. In the group, you may rehearse interactions with others that you think might be difficult for you. This rehearsal helps you prepare for a difficult situation, and possibly prevent a negative outcome. To help you keep a more positive and realistic view of yourself, you might be asked to list your positive traits or characteristics. While it may be difficult for you to think positively about yourself, it is important to your personhood to focus on the positive aspects of who you are. When you start listing your positive qualities, you will be more easily reminded that you have a number of good traits. I often suggest that people with memory loss keep that list close to them; to carry it in their pocket book or purse as a reminder of the good qualities they possess. Then, when you tend to overgeneralize or blame yourself when things go wrong, you will have a positive reminder of your good qualities to balance any negative feelings about yourself.

If you are interested in being part of a cognitive-behavioral therapy group, your healthcare provider may refer you to a professional who conducts these therapies. Cognitive-behavioral therapies can be especially helpful as you adjust to the disease diagnosis and changing abilities. One note here: some healthcare providers *mistakenly* believe that individuals with progressive memory loss or dementia cannot benefit from this therapy or that insurance programs, such as Medicare, will not help pay for this therapy. A qualified therapist will inform you if you cannot benefit from cognitive-behavioral therapy. You or your family member should ask for an evaluation by a therapist before allowing anyone to conclude that you cannot benefit from it.

Setting yourself up for success

Another approach to maintaining personhood and decreasing negative feelings is to arrange interactions and social situations so the best outcome will result. When you think about the social situations in which you will take part, identify the demands that these situations make on you. Once you realize what a situation might require, you can then arrange to take part in interactions in a positive way. For example, if you have difficulty following a conversation when there are several people talking at the same time, you may want to avoid being part of a large group of people. Instead, look for small groups of only one or two people and join a small group for conversation. In this way, you are more likely to follow the conversation and respond appropriately. If you are afraid you will forget names, write the names of the people you know will be present at a social event on a piece of paper before the event. Keep the paper in your pocket or purse to help you recall a person's name. You can also identify social situations that involve activities in which you will do well. For example, many people with memory loss have played bridge all of their life. With memory loss, playing such a complicated game may be a challenge for you. If playing a card game is important to you as a person, however, you may want to join a different group that plays a less complicated card game. Setting yourself up for success allows you to continue activities that define your personhood. If success is more likely to occur, you will protect yourself from negative feelings. A number of different ways are possible to help ensure success, depending upon your strengths and the activities essential to your personhood.

Validating interactions

A therapist named Naomi Feil (1993) developed an approach to interacting with people with memory loss called "validation." Using this approach, interactions center on understanding the meaning behind the words and actions of individuals with memory loss. Often, family members and friends tend to correct a mistake or point out errors in your words or actions. With validation, instead of correcting you, a family member might instead say something like, "I know it is hard for you to find the right words when you feel rushed. It's OK to take your time. We want to hear what you have to say." This type of validating response lets you know that you are understood—and accepted. Validation allows you the freedom to be yourself in an interaction. The person with whom you are interacting also has the benefit of learning more about you by giving you the chance to express your thoughts and feelings. Validating interactions require the other person to understand the process and be willing to use this positive method of interacting. Close and loving people in your life may welcome the chance to learn about this positive way of interacting once they understand the benefit for both themselves and you. Validating interactions can help you keep a sense of personhood and create positive feelings—outcomes that are well worth the effort needed to learn how to use this positive way of interacting.

Maintaining relationships

Early in this chapter, personhood was defined as including relationships with others. Keeping important and close relationships alive and positive can help maintain your own personhood. Positive relationships provide you with comfort and reassurance. Comfort carries with it a sense of closeness. Comfort can ease the initial distress that occurs with a diagnosis of progressive memory loss. Close and positive relationships also provide you with a sense of attachment to others. The need for attachment is universal. We all need to be part of a larger group: a family, a friendship, or social network that has meaning to your personhood. Continuing these relationships is a very powerful way to support who you are as a person. Close relationships can be reassuring as you go through changes caused by progressive memory loss. Relationships provide a safety net for some of the losses that you might experience. A sense of inclusion is also part of relationships. With any disease, continuing to feel a part of everyday activities provides positive support for your personhood—to be included in a way consistent with your past. When this need for inclusion is met, your sense of who you are as a person is easier to maintain as you identify with your place in the group.

Strategies for keeping positive relationships are described in a later chapter in this book. The importance of relationships to your personhood is mentioned here to help you be aware of how essential relationships are to maintaining personhood. Your ability to love and care for others is a valued part of yourself that will need to be expressed throughout your disease.

Final thoughts

The process of growing older results in every older adult being unique. The process of progressive memory loss is also unique for every person. However, some common needs exist for those with progressive memory loss. We began this chapter by describing how Thomas Kitwood (1997a, 1997b) defines personhood. Dr. Kitwood also described the basic needs of people with progressive memory loss. Meeting these basic needs will assist you in keeping a positive and enduring sense of personhood. The six basic needs described by Dr. Kitwood include the following.

1. *Attachment*: Attachment includes a sense of belonging and forming strong bonds with others. Attachments provide a safety net for people with progressive memory loss and allow you to function at your best.

2. *Inclusion*: Each person with progressive memory loss continues to need to be part of a larger group. Being part of a group allows you to relate to others, expand and grow, and to combat the loneliness that often goes along with memory loss.

3. *Occupation*: Even in the presence of progressive memory loss, people need to be engaged in activities that are worthwhile and rewarding. Activities that were rewarding or positive in the past continue to be a valued part of your life. Activities can involve both work and play. The important aspect of occupation is being engaged in a way that decreases boredom and the desire to withdraw.

4. *Identity*: Your identity includes both the present (who you are now) and a sense of continuity with the past. Others support your identity. You also have your own sense of who you are and what is important in your life. Your sense of identity helps you recognize how you are unique as a person.

5. *Comfort*: Comfort is essential for providing the strength and feelings of security we need when faced with progressive memory

loss. Comfort can help you deal with the everyday anxieties that often go along with the changes you may experience. Comfort can be found in closeness with others and the caring they provide. Comfort can also be found in knowing who you are and keeping a sense of your self alive and well.

6. *Love:* The final need of individuals with progressive memory loss is love. This need can be fulfilled in part by meeting the other needs described above. Love given to you allows you to feel valued and have a general sense of self-worth. Love that you share with others gives meaning to your life and increases your self-worth. This sense of self-worth will support your personhood in positive ways.

These basic needs are the same for all people, with or without progressive memory loss. The interventions and actions we have described in this chapter will assist you in meeting these basic needs. As your needs are met, your self-perceptions will be more positive. Your sense of personhood will also be maintained at higher levels. An enduring sense of personhood will provide meaning and support as you manage the effects of progressive memory loss. A simple guide to staying in touch with your personhood is found at the end of this chapter. You may use this guide to remind you daily of the ways you can stay positive about who you are as a person.

STRATEGIES TO HELP YOU MAINTAIN YOUR SENSE OF PERSONHOOD

- Avoid being negative about yourself.
- Avoid all-or-nothing thinking, such as, "If I do one thing wrong, I am a bad person."
- Avoid blaming yourself for things you cannot control.
- Stay active and involved with positive activities.
- Set yourself up for success. Design activities based on your abilities.
- Use validating communications to help others understand the meaning behind your words and actions.
- Keep important and close relationships alive and positive.
- Meet your basic needs for:
  - being attached to others
  - staying occupied or productive
  - being included in groups and conversations
  - being aware of who you are as a person
  - comfort through close relationships
  - loving relationships.

CHAPTER 3

Maintaining Important
Roles in Your Life

Role changes are common in any progressive illness that impairs thinking and memory. Although some of your abilities may be altered, most of your roles will still be important to your sense of self. In my work with people with Alzheimer's disease, one of the questions I would routinely ask the person with memory loss was, "How would you best describe yourself today?" Almost every person with memory loss would describe themselves by roles they had filled previously, such as "mother," "farmer," "banker," and so forth. These roles served as their identity—much more than physical appearance ("I'm tall and grey-haired") or personality characteristics ("I'm happy and positive"). Rarely did the person describe him- or herself in any terms other than the roles they had filled much of their lives. These responses speak of the importance of roles to each person, even with changes in mental ability and memory loss. The roles you have assumed previously or might continue are closely tied to your sense of who you are.

The important roles in your life also help you have a continuous link to your past. Having this connection to your past can help maintain memory and a sense of who you are. For example, if you have always been a favorite aunt or uncle, your relatives will always recall how you functioned as aunt or uncle. They will continue to see you in this role, based on how you have lived it in the past. Roles also help define how you continue to relate to others. How you have fulfilled your role as a parent, for example, may define how you continue to interact with your children. For instance, if you provided guidance for your children much of their lives, they may continue to look to you for advice concerning major life decisions. If your role as parent was more supportive, your children may continue to expect that support. Your role in the workplace defined how you related to your co-workers and colleagues. If you were a supervisor or assumed a management role, your colleagues will look to you for direction and support. Maintaining your roles directly affects your ability to maintain your personhood, the connection to your past, and how you will continue to relate to others.

Generally, roles are arranged or defined with others. For instance, in the past you may have been responsible for managing your family's finances. This role was probably agreeable to your spouse. With memory loss, you may find some parts of this role becoming more difficult to fill. You may want to continue in this role, yet your spouse may have a different opinion. You and your spouse will need to talk about this role and agree on how you will continue to assist with finances. Coming to this agreement about changes in role often requires you to work out the agreement with other people involved in that role.

Roles depend upon relationships. For example, a leader needs a follower and a cook needs someone to eat the food. This need to talk about and agree on role changes with others may seem threatening to you at times. For some, the process of reaching an agreement allows a person to function at the highest level possible in the role. For others, the outcomes may be less positive, especially if everyone involved in the relationship does not agree on the best way for you to continue in a role. In my work, I have seen a lack of agreement occur most often in regards to the role of driver. Many people with progressive memory loss may still feel comfortable being the driver of the family car—a role they might have filled most of their adult life. But, a spouse or other family members may not agree. The final agreement about the driver role may not always result in the person with memory loss continuing to be the primary driver for the family. The result is less participation in the driver role than you really want. The following example of an outcome of less participation is very typical.

Harry's story

Harry, a very intelligent 80-year-old retired engineer, would often express his frustration with role changes. During each visit together, over several years, Harry would comment to me, "She [his wife] doesn't even allow me to make mistakes any more. I know I can't do everything as well as I used to, but I would like to at least have the chance to try. I would like to be allowed to make a mistake at least once in a while."

Maintaining the role you want requires an honest appraisal of yourself and coming to terms with the abilities or strengths that you continue to possess. Role change also includes a thoughtful consideration of what this change means to others involved in the role. You might want to consider the following helpful ways to continue in the roles you have had in the past.

Attempt to focus on the positive

What parts of the role provide you with the greatest joy and personal satisfaction? How can your continued participation in the role benefit others? For example, if you have been the financial manager in the family, what aspects of this role do you really enjoy? Reading the financial pages of the newspaper? Writing the checks to pay the bills? Balancing the checkbook? Try to identify the part of the role that you care about the most. Also, consider how your continuing in that part of the role will help others. Will your participation in decisions about finances take pressure off of your spouse? Can you offer advice to your spouse based on what you read in the financial news? Identifying the benefits of continuing in parts of the role will help you see how you can change or narrow the role in a way that is positive for everyone.

Act on your own behalf

You will need to act on your own behalf in talking about role change. This may seem difficult to you, considering the changes you are experiencing. How can you be sure others will listen and respect you when you tell them what you want to happen? You may not be sure that anyone will listen to you, but if you do not talk to others and express what you want, no one *can* listen. Sometimes, friends and family members may make these decisions for you—not out of disrespect—but simply because they do not know your wishes. Expressing your wishes about continuing in your roles in a positive and realistic way will help others hear your wishes. When expressing your wishes, try starting your sentences with the word "I." For example, "I would like to continue to see all of the bills." "I would like to be part of all discussions about money with the children." Try to avoid beginning your sentences with the word "You." These sentences often sound accusatory. For example, "You never let me decide anything anymore." By using "I" statements, you are asserting yourself in a positive way—you are also more likely to be heard.

The negative effects of not acting on your own behalf can be found in the following true example.

Mildred's story

Mildred was an exceptionally intelligent member of a support group I directed for people with memory loss. She had never married and spent most of her adult years teaching in secondary education. She had served as an expert in her field most of her life. At one support group meeting, Mildred stated, with some grief, "No one asks me questions any more. I really miss being the person others come to for advice." In talking about this very real concern, Mildred said that she had never told others about her need to continue to be a resource and expert in her field. Mildred was certainly able to provide guidance and information to others—she was just not able to speak on her own behalf. She was unable to let others know of her desire to continue in this lifelong role. As a result, Mildred withdrew from an important part of her previous role long before she lost the ability to fill the role.

Be honest with yourself

Try to be as objective as possible about the role and your ability to fill the role. This can hard for you, as you will tend to see yourself as you always have. You may find it difficult to see how the changes inherent in progressive memory loss are affecting your ability to function in a role you have done most of your life. It may take many months or even years for you to change how you view yourself. This slow change in how you view yourself makes it very hard for you to be objective about your abilities. You may also feel hurt when others suggest that a role that used to be easy may now be too difficult for you. Often, family members and friends focus primarily on the things you *cannot* do any longer. You need to call attention to the things you still can do. Try to identify some of the abilities you have that are needed to fill the role. For example, you could say something like, "I can still write checks." You could also admit something like, "I just can't balance the checkbook anymore." Being honest with yourself and others will help others recognize that you are aware of both your abilities and limits.

The following examples are true stories of individuals with progressive memory loss. The first story describes a man, Frank, who was able to keep many of his previous roles. The second story is about a woman, Ruth, who gave up many of her previous roles well before she was unable to continue filling them. In Frank's story, you will find positive ways to maintain roles. Ruth's story, on the other hand, gives you examples of actions you will want to avoid.

Frank's story

Frank, a man in his mid-sixties, was diagnosed with Alzheimer's disease. Frank was highly successful, launching his own company at a young age. For most of his adult life, Frank served as a chief executive officer (CEO) for that company. In this role, Frank supervised all of his employees and directed the everyday business of this company. When Frank was diagnosed with Alzheimer's disease, he was still active in his CEO role. Frank's role in the company was so important to him that he did not want to give up all the tasks he had taken on over the years. Frank and his wife together were able to find parts of the CEO role that Frank could continue to fill. They were also able to find new tasks Frank could assume within the company that fitted in with his abilities. Frank's wife worked with the staff at his office to design activities that Frank could do even when he was not able to manage the company's finances. Also, Frank shortened his daily time at the office from a full day to about three hours in the morning. No longer able to drive, Frank walked to work each day (about a half-mile from his home), spent the morning at the office, and walked home at noon. For about two years after Frank's diagnosis, he was able to continue to walk to and from work every day and do parts of his previous role. By being honest about his abilities, Frank was able to work with his wife and co-workers to find tasks that he enjoyed and was able to do. Together, they found a way for Frank to work in the company that he loved. This continued role, although changed from what Frank had done before, gave Frank satisfaction and helped keep him both mentally and physically active.

The positive results from Frank's role change would not have happened if Frank had not been willing to act on his own behalf. Frank was able to let his wife and co-workers know about his desire to continue managing the company. If Frank had not expressed his wishes, his wife and colleagues may have assumed he was ready to retire. Frank was also willing and able to be objective about his abilities. The role he assumed after his diagnosis did not include all of Frank's previous tasks. Frank was able to see for himself that he needed to work a shorter day. He also accepted the need to turn over much of the financial management to someone else. Frank continued to have a positive view of changes in his role, even talking about the benefits of walking to work—rather than being upset about the loss of his driving abilities. Throughout the two years Frank continued in this changed role, he often spoke of the joy he received in working at his company. Just being in the office where Frank had spent so many years of his life was rewarding and positive for everyone, including Frank's family.

Ruth's story

Ruth was the wife of a very public figure in a large community. In her role, Ruth had become well known in the community because her husband's work required her to appear in public with him. Ruth was an active member and leader of many committees. She also assisted with social events associated with her husband's work. Ruth was diagnosed with Alzheimer's disease in her early sixties—a time when her husband was at the peak of his career. The news about Ruth's diagnosis spread quickly across the couple's large social network. The response to the news about Ruth's diagnosis was an outpouring of help from friends and family members. What friends and family members did not understand, however, was the need to allow Ruth to continue in her previous roles. Friends just took over many of the roles Ruth had done before her diagnosis. Friends started bringing over food nightly so Ruth would not need to prepare meals. At one point, Ruth said, "When I open the door in the afternoon and see someone standing there with food in their hands, I sometimes just want to slam the door and tell them to 'go away'. I want to cook for my husband. I don't want others taking over for me." This help from others did not allow Ruth to do the things that she loved. In this true example, Ruth's ability to continue to function in her previous roles was hampered by some very well-meaning friends and family members. The result of this help was negative for Ruth. She was depressed during much of the first few years after her diagnosis. Ruth felt as if she had no control over the limits that were placed on her role as wife and these limits added to her depression.

Several things added to this negative outcome for Ruth. First, Ruth said that she did not feel comfortable acting on her own behalf. She had always taken a back seat to her husband, and she just could not assert herself and express her needs after her diagnosis. Ruth had spent many of her adult years supporting her husband's work. She always placed his needs before her own, and this added to a more negative outcome. No family member or friend took the time to talk with Ruth about her needs. No one asked Ruth about what she was able to continue doing and what she wanted to do. No one took the time to find ways to change Ruth's roles so that she could continue to do some parts of the role. The result was that Ruth gave up many of her roles well before she needed too. Ruth could have continued to do many of her roles as housekeeper, expert cook, and community leader had the roles been changed to match her abilities. For instance, Ruth was able to cook one dish long after she was not able to prepare a whole meal. Ruth could have added to social events by bringing a dish to share even after she was not able to host an entire event or meeting. The changes in Ruth's roles forced on to her by others resulted in Ruth becoming isolated, angry, and sad. These negative outcomes for Ruth could have been prevented if she had taken part in deciding how and when her roles would change. Also, Ruth could have stayed more active in her roles if family members and friends had taken the time to change the role to match her abilities.

Results of role changes

The roles that you give up may be the most important to your continued functioning and independence. Often the role of provider for the family is one of the first roles that is lost, as you may not be able to continue to work. For women, the role of housekeeper is a traditional role for much of their lives. Early in memory loss, family members and paid assistants often take over this role. You may want and may be able to do some part of the role if it is changed to match your abilities. When you stop a role, the role is often taken over by someone else. One way to prevent a total loss of roles is to help you find ways to continue in some of your previous roles. Your family members and friends also need to understand your need to continue in a role to the fullest extent possible.

Keeping some part of your previous roles is important for several reasons. First, the loss of a role can result in a lowered sense of personhood—or who you are. Your hopes for the future are often tied to your ability to fill previous roles. If you know you will still be "father," "grandma," "gardener," "artist," or "teacher," you will be more positive about your future. You will also have a stronger sense of who you are as you face changes in memory and mental abilities. Second, giving up important roles may keep you from taking part in activities you enjoy. You may become isolated from friends and others you value. In a study of people diagnosed with progressive memory loss (mostly Alzheimer's disease), one of the strongest influences on quality of life was the degree to which the individuals stayed involved in activities they had previously enjoyed. Continuing in your previous roles may help you stay active and involved, resulting in a higher quality of life.

Giving up an important role may also increase negative moods or depression. If you do not feel productive or useful, these negative feelings can result in negative moods or depression. Depression is especially a concern right after you receive a diagnosis—a time during which you may be still be active in your previous roles. Continuing in your previous roles may help battle the negative moods that are common after a diagnosis of progressive memory loss. Lastly, giving up roles can result in feelings of being powerless, with little control over your life. If you do not have a voice in how your roles change, you may feel as if you have lost control over parts of your life that are important to you. This loss of control may increase your feelings of being powerless. The following suggestions may help you find ways to change your previous roles to help you continue in a way that is positive and meaningful.

Ways to maintain previous roles
Get help from others
Family members and friends can give you help to stay in a previous role. Giving help means that others are willing to be supportive and to help you find ways to meet your needs. In the work setting, this help may happen when someone identifies parts of your role that match the abilities you have retained. For instance, you may not be able to direct a project any more. But, you may be able to give helpful advice. Changing your role from a project director to a team member will help you stay in some part of the role.

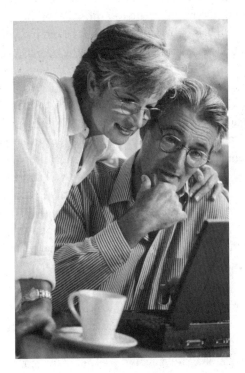

Help to stay in a role may happen just by changing the speed of actions and your responses. It takes longer for people with memory loss to process information and respond. Your family members, co-workers, and friends can make it easier for you to stay in a role by just slowing down the speed of your conversation and tasks. Allowing more time to process information allows you to understand what is being asked of you. When you have time to respond, you are more likely to give a correct response. In the home, your role can also be made easier in much the same way. For example, it may take you longer to remember everything you need to plant a garden or pay the bills. However, if you are given more time to remember or even make a list, then you will probably be able to complete the tasks necessary for that role. Slowing down the speed of tasks and giving you more time to complete each one is a way others can help you stay active in a previous role.

Sharing a role

A second way to keep part of an important role is to share the role with someone else. This reminds me of the old saying, "Two heads are better than one." In the work setting, parts of the role that fit with your retained abilities can be continued. The parts of the role that are too difficult can be given to the person with whom you are sharing the role. At work, for example, you may still be able to take inventory and place orders, but the monthly expense reports may be too difficult for you to complete. By sharing that part of your work role, preparing the monthly reports, with someone else, the entire role can be done with success. This type of role-sharing is common in the work setting. You can also use role-sharing outside of work. In a housekeeping role, you may want to share some of the difficult tasks with a home assistant. For example, it may be hard for you to plan an entire meal, but by sharing meal preparation with a home assistant, you may prepare parts of the meal. Or, you and a family member or friend may have a "cooking day" and make several meals ahead to freeze and reheat during the week. Many busy young mothers use this very same method. One advantage of using role-sharing is that you will be able to stay active in the role. Also, the skills and knowledge you bring to that role will be seen in the positive outcomes.

Make a new role

At times, you may need to construct a new role to keep it as part of your life. New roles can be made by changing your expectations of yourself. When you change your expectations, you may find yourself making a role easier or simplifying it in a way that makes it possible for you. Making a role easier or different is one of the most widely used and practical ways to stay in a role. This reminds me of the old saying about how "less" can really be "more." One reason individuals with memory loss often give for not keeping a previous role is fear of failure and embarrassment. By making a new role easier than the old role, success can be increased. Your fear of failure will no longer keep you from staying active in the role.

Making a role easier can be used for almost any role, including work. One example of the positive benefits of making a role easier can be found in a true story of a very talented woman, Linda, who was diagnosed with Alzheimer's disease in her mid-sixties. Linda's career was playing professional golf for most of her adult life. She reached a point when she was not able to play a full round of 18 holes. When this happened, Linda gave up golf, even though "golfer" was a major role in her life. When I first met Linda, she was depressed, withdrawn, and negative about her future. After talking with Linda and her family over several months, we were able to design a putting green for her in her backyard. Linda's family also started taking her to the driving range, where she could continue to practice golf. Even though Linda could not play 18 holes of golf, she was able to go out in her backyard and continue in her previous role. By making golf easier, she could stay active in a lifelong role. The result for Linda was positive. Linda had an immediate increase in physical activity, her depression lessened, and she had a more positive outlook about her future.

Almost any role can be made easier to allow you to continue in the role. A farmer may not be able to plant a field of corn, but may be able to help with harvest, to take the harvest to market, and help with the decisions that go along with farming. A carpenter may not be able to operate complicated power tools, but may be able to sand wood, glue parts together, and apply finishes. A housekeeper may not be able to go to the grocery store by herself, but may be able to use a list to buy groceries and put them away once she is home. You can see that almost any role can be altered to allow you to continue in the role. By making the role easier, you will have less fear of failure. You will be setting yourself up for success. The more you succeed in the role, the more likely you are to continue to stay in the role. Family members, friends, and co-workers can all help find ways to fit the role to your abilities. The results will be positive for everyone.

Maintaining roles within the family

Relationships or "feeling connected to others" are important to staying in a role. Paying attention to being connected to others is somewhat like the saying, "It's not what you know, it's who you know." I think that this saying is often true for people with memory loss. The work of Lisa Snyder (2002) and others supports the reality of a basic need of individuals with memory loss to be connected to others. This need is part of your need for companionship, the need to feel valued, and the sense of belonging to a larger social group. You will also need others to have meaningful and stimulating activities. Those with memory loss may have a harder time meeting this need. Why? Some of your family members and friends may think (wrongly) that your memory problems mean you don't need a relationship anymore. Some people, even close family members and friends, may be afraid that they will say the wrong thing to you. This causes them to just not say anything at all! This lack of communication can make it very difficult for you to feel connected with others. In interviews with 60 people with Alzheimer's disease, Dr. Snyder found that individuals with the disease had major concerns about their relationships with family members and friends. Those with memory loss had fears of becoming dependent on others. They also feared that family members would insist on changes in their roles. People with memory loss knew that it was necessary for family members to want to work with them for the relationships to be positive. They feared that family members would not always be willing to work with them. These concerns may not be the same for everyone with memory loss. However, these concerns are common in situations where one person in the relationship faces a change in abilities. The following section describes actions you may use to help manage your concerns about changes in roles that involve relationships with others.

Roles in marriage

In families, roles may include the role of husband or wife within a marriage. Within the marriage, a variety of roles may occur: lover, financial manager, household manager, activity planner, and so on. Many of these roles may have defined how you and your spouse relate to each other on a daily basis. These roles may also define how you relate to others outside of the marriage. For instance, if you have been the person to plan each family gathering, a change in this role will affect your spouse—and other family members. Therefore, changes in a role within the marriage may have a ripple effect, affecting how you relate to others outside your marriage.

Research with people with memory loss has shown how much they value the companionship and intimacy in their marriage. Individuals clearly described how much they wanted to continue an intimate relationship with their spouse. Those with memory loss, however, often described loss of intimacy as a common change in the marriage. In my interviews, one gentleman in his early seventies often said, "You know, she moved out of our bedroom, and that really hurt. I'm not ready to stop sleeping with my wife, but she didn't even ask if I wanted her to move out." This type of change in intimacy with a lifelong partner may be hurtful to you—and it is often not necessary. This change in your role as a marriage partner may also happen without your agreement. The loss of intimacy might leave you wondering if you have done something wrong. You might even fear that your partner is having an affair or is planning a divorce. Your spouse, on the other hand, might think that this change is not important to you. Your spouse may make this decision without knowing that you want to be part of any decisions that are made about your marriage, including sleeping arrangements. Your spouse may have good intentions and may not understand that this change in intimacy is hurtful to you. In this situation, you may need to speak for yourself, using a sentence beginning with "I." For example, "I would like to keep sleeping together." By making your wishes known to your spouse, you can help your spouse understand that you do care about your marriage. You can also decrease the risk that a change will happen without your voice being heard.

Sexual intimacy or closeness may be a hard part of your marriage to talk about. Some individuals, particularly men, have an increase in their need for sexual contact, although this also happens in women. This hypersexuality or increased need for sexual contact is hard for the person with memory loss to understand and may also be misunderstood by the spouse. This behavior in men is often viewed negatively: just being a "dirty old man." It may also be threatening to a spouse if sexual overtones are expressed to other women, something that occurs in men with progressive memory loss. You may not even be aware of this change in your behavior or sexual needs, so you may not see the need to talk about this behavior with your spouse. On the other hand, some spouses are not sure if the spouse with memory loss shares their desire for sexual contact and intimacy. The husband or wife may feel guilty if they want sexual contact and intimacy and the spouse with memory loss does not respond to that desire positively. You can see how this confusion about sexual contact and intimacy can cause problems or loss of intimacy in a marriage. If this happens in your marriage, an open and honest talk with your spouse may be helpful. This might also be the time to ask for advice from an outside expert: a counselor or pastor with some experience in marital counseling. Knowing that changes in sexual intimacy and sex drive can happen with memory loss is one step to preventing even greater problems. An open discussion, counseling, or both may help you to retain sexual intimacy as long as possible in your marriage.

Throughout the years, people with memory loss and their spouses have told me about some very creative, yet simple, ways to help keep marriage roles alive and positive for both partners. Over and over, both the person with memory loss and their spouse have described the many rewards of keeping marriage roles. One approach to keeping a role in a marriage is to break down the different parts of the marriage. You and your spouse can look at what makes your marriage work. Even something as simple as being the person to pay the bill when shopping or eating a meal away from home can help a marriage function without losses to the person with memory loss. One very sensitive wife described how she would provide her husband, diagnosed with Alzheimer's disease in his early fifties, with just enough money to pay for a meal prior to leaving the home when his ability to calculate the correct change became impaired. By using his previous role in the marriage, this simple act by the wife allowed her husband to continue in his role as bill payer within their marriage. Helping the husband keep this part of his marriage role protected his self-esteem. Helping him to perform this role also kept that part of their marriage (eating out with family members and friends) alive and positive for them both.

One very loving husband also found small ways to keep his marriage alive. In this example, the couple had a lifelong habit of sitting together every night after dinner and watching the news together. His wife, who had been diagnosed with Alzheimer's disease for a number of years, was often unable to sit for a long periods of time. To keep an important part of the marriage, every evening the husband would take his wife's hand, go to their chairs in the living room, and watch the news together. He would talk with her about the news, making sure he gave her enough time to respond. For both, this time together became one of the most meaningful and peaceful times of the day. Because this was one part of their lifelong marriage, this simple act of sitting together every evening kept an important part of their marriage roles alive. These examples are just a few of the many ways you and your spouse can sustain the roles important to your marriage. By finding simple ways to keep these roles in your marriage alive, both you and your spouse can keep your marriage positive and fulfilling.

Family relationships

Within your family, you may have many roles: parent, sibling, or grandparent. You can continue in these roles even though you have memory loss. Sometimes fear of failing may cause you to avoid family activities. It is important to recognize and manage your fears to keep an active role in your family. This type of fear may be similar to what Franklin Delano Roosevelt meant when he said after Pearl Harbor, "We have nothing to fear but fear itself!" One very independent 70-year-old widow I knew, Mabel, lived in an assisted living facility. Mabel loved her daughter and grandchildren dearly, but feared she would say something wrong in front of the grandchildren. Her daughter would bring the grandchildren to visit, but Mabel refused to go out to family events or gatherings. She eventually spent less and less time with her grandchildren, because of her fears. Mabel lost these valued family relationships and missed time with her family. This change in the family relationship was not necessary and Mabel's grandchildren were deprived of the cherished time they could have spent with her.

Again, people with memory loss and their family members have shared with me many examples of successful ways to keep family roles alive and well. One father–daughter pair was very creative in the how they kept their relationship alive. First, they agreed that when the father made a mistake they would both do their best not to take the error to heart, but instead often laughed at the mistake. The father would sometimes forget to put on socks with his shoes or would have mismatched socks—a simple mistake, but sometimes embarrassing if it would happen in public. When this happened, the daughter would often say something like, "Dad, you did it again! Look at those socks!" Then, they would both have a good laugh and correct the mistake together. This honest way of dealing with common mistakes prevented something else that can occur in families: role reversal. By talking about the mistake in a non-threatening way and solving the problem together, the daughter allowed her father to act as independently as possible. She also kept herself from assuming a caregiver role. This creative father–daughter pair also kept their relationship alive in other ways. The father with memory loss was very physically active and was an avid bicyclist. To spend quality time together, the pair agreed to bicycle together two to three times a week. After work, the daughter and father would go on long bike rides. During this time, they talked about family matters, his memory loss, and how he was managing day-to-day challenges. For several years, this time together helped to maintain the daughter's relationship with her father. This private time also allowed the father to talk about his disease in a safe, accepting way. The exercise gave them both physical and mental benefits as well. This planned activity helped the father keep his role as advisor for his daughter—a role he had always valued. What a simple, positive way to a positive outcome for everyone!

When thinking about your family members and the relationships you have now, you may decide on the roles you want the keep. You may then find ways to keep those roles and relationships as intact as possible. Each person's relationship with their children and grandchildren is different, of course. Each relationship has activities and roles that are important to you and the other person. You might try asking yourself the following questions to help you decide how best to keep these activities as part of your role. If you are a grandparent, what types of activities with your grandchildren give you the greatest satisfaction and enjoyment? Are these activities enjoyable for your grandchildren as well? How can these activities and roles be made easier so that you can continue them in a positive way without a fear of failing? How can your abilities be used to fill your role as a parent and grandparent for as long as possible? One grandmother told me how, after she was unable to drive, she would meet her granddaughter at the bus stop each day to walk her home after school. She used this time to talk with her granddaughter about her day, giving her granddaughter support while helping to keep the relationship positive. Rather than giving up this time with her granddaughter when she was not able to drive, this creative grandmother found a way to continue her role without fear of failing herself or her granddaughter. Answering these questions for yourself and focusing on the things you are still able to do will help you find activities to keep your valued family relationships.

Friendships and community relationships

Maintaining previous roles with friends may present some challenges for individuals with memory loss. Much like a marriage, each friendship is unique. Some friendships center on previous work roles, some on social groups (dance, community, civic), and some on faith-based activities, such as church groups. Some friends may seem more uncomfortable around you once they learn about your diagnosis. Others will continue to treat you in the same way as they have in the past. These responses from friends may help you decide which friendships you will keep and which friendships may no longer be positive for you.

People with memory loss often describe instances of lost friendships, even when the friendship has been established for a long time. One couple took part in a weekly exercise program I was conducting. The wife, Mary, was diagnosed with Alzheimer's disease in her late fifties. While Mary was usually very happy and pleasant, one day she was obviously "down" during one of our walks together. When I asked both Mary and her husband, John, about the change in her mood, they told me about an incident that occurred the previous weekend. For over 20 years, this couple had an arrangement with four other couples to meet and eat together every Friday evening. Without any known reason, the previous Friday evening John and Mary were not invited to eat dinner with the other four couples. They learned later that the other couples had, in fact, continued their tradition and had eaten together. The other couples had evidently chosen not to include John and Mary in this group any longer. This change in a valued friendship was obviously hurtful to both John and Mary. Through no action or choice on their part, John and Mary were excluded from an important part of their social life and friendships. This type of pulling away by previous friends and social groups has been described as a frequent outcome of progressive memory loss. While painful, this pulling away can help you learn about the friends whom you can depend on and will want to keep in your life. Reaching this understanding about who are your true friends may be painful at first, but may result in less distress and more positive results over time.

Once true friendships are evident, the process of redefining your role in the friendship can begin. You may decide there are parts of each friendship that you want to keep. Many people with progressive memory loss are members of professional groups, such as Kiwanis, the Optimist Club, or Rotary. These friendships and groups often represent lifelong ties and valued social events. Although you may not be able to drive to these meetings or take a leadership role, you may still participate and keep the friendships. Friends and other club members may help you by providing transport to meetings. The pace of the meetings may be slowed down to allow you to follow what is being said and acted upon. Making these simple changes in these friendship groups allows you to continue with the friendships in a way that is positive for you.

Friends in faith-based groups, such as churches and synagogues, are often very willing to help find ways to keep you active and participating. Accepting help from friends in a faith-based group may be hard at first, as you might have been the one to provide help in the past. As one person expressed, "I have been a member of that church for over 30 years and have assisted others many times. I understand that someone may want to help me now." Learning to feel comfortable with this change in your role and being willing to accept help may be the key to staying active in your role in a faith-based group. The changes needed to help stay in a role vary with the role. For example, one choir member with memory loss had trouble learning new songs and reading some of the lyrics quickly. To help her stay in the choir, the choir director would often choose songs that were familiar. The person with memory loss could sing from memory and felt good about continuing to be part of the choir. Another person with memory loss had played the organ for her church for many years. When she no longer felt comfortable playing alone in front of the entire congregation, she would assist the new organist and accompany the choir during rehearsals. Many simple changes can be made in how you participate in a faith-based group to allow you to continue in your previous roles.

Community roles

In a personal description of the effects of memory loss, Henderson says, "Sometimes we miss being important—miss being needed (1998, p.36). Community roles are often roles that fill this need to be needed—to continue to be productive in society. Community roles, along with work roles, are also some of the first roles that are dropped or changed after a diagnosis of progressive memory loss. Fear of failure or embarrassment may result in you giving up community roles in which you have previously served—often before this is necessary. You may be able to continue in certain parts of community roles by focussing on the abilities you still have. Changing a previous community role may be more positive than giving up the role entirely and losing that part of your sense of self.

Serving as a volunteer is one way to act on your values regarding your role in society and your need to contribute in a meaningful way. Taking part in a voluntary activity contributes to your feelings of being productive, successful, and a competent person. Even at times of critical life events, such as a diagnosis of progressive memory loss, volunteer roles can lessen some of the stress that goes along with such a diagnosis. Some community groups have developed volunteer programs just for people with progressive memory loss, such as Alzheimer's disease. These programs have placed individuals in volunteer positions matched to their level of retained ability. Volunteer positions include a wide range of activities, such as working at a natural history museum, assisting with a children's reading program, assisting with mailings at the local Alzheimer's Association, working in homeless shelters, and working in the Salvation Army resale shops. These activities provide positive benefits for each group. The volunteer activities also give you the chance to fulfill your need to contribute to society. This win–win situation can happen in any community. If being a volunteer has been important to you in the past, it may be important for you to seek out "safe" volunteer roles in your community. To ensure success, ask about all the tasks involved in any volunteer role to make sure the tasks fit with your abilities. You might also want to enlist a friend or family member to take part in the volunteer program with you, to provide you with support if needed. Most important, having a diagnosis of progressive memory loss does not mean that you need to give up the role of volunteer, especially if it has been a rewarding part of your life.

What next?

The loss of previous roles can result in negative outcomes for you. Role change and loss can cause feelings of being powerless, withdrawal from social groups, loss of closeness or intimacy in a marriage or family relationship, and increases in negative mood or depression. Importantly, changing your role may help you function in the role as long as possible. Continuing to perform a role may have long-term positive effects on your physical, mental, and emotional wellbeing. Maintaining previous roles will also help you to keep your sense of self. You can help to continue your previous roles by focusing on the positive parts of the role, acting on your own behalf, and being honest about your abilities. Others can help you stay in a role by assisting you, sharing the role with you, and making the role easier. Acting on your own behalf, you may let others know you need to change the role and to slow the speed of tasks and discussions to allow you to understand and respond correctly. Making sure the role matches your abilities will help you have success and reduce your fear of failing. No single approach to changing your role will be successful every time. However, trying different ways to change the role makes it more likely that you will be able to stay in the role.

Roles occur in a marriage, in families, and with friends. Each role may be changed to allow you to function at your best. Working with your spouse and other family members will help you find ways to keep these roles alive. At other times, you will need to act on your own behalf. The need to act on your own behalf may be more difficult if you find you are not heard by others. Family members, friends, and co-workers may not be sensitive to and aware of your need to be heard. They may also find it difficult to understand how important your roles are to you. You may not always be given the chance to express your wishes. Helping others to understand your concerns and your need to continue to be yourself may be one of the most important things you can do for yourself. Often, people with progressive memory loss have said the most important thing to them is to be "treated like they have always been treated." The suggestions in this chapter may help you meet the need to be who you have always been and fill the roles that are important to you. You can use the journal at the end of this chapter to outline the roles you want to maintain. You can then decide what actions you want to take to allow you to continue in the role.

SAMPLE ROLE MAINTENANCE JOURNAL

Role	Steps to stay active in role	Ability
Example: Church organist	1. Select music that is familiar.	Can read music
	2. Play only one or two hymns each service.	
	3. Have someone help turn the pages of the music.	Can concentrate well on one thing at a time.
	4. Play only for morning services.	Most alert in morning.

YOUR ROLE MAINTENANCE JOURNAL

Role	Steps to stay active in role	Ability
1.	1.	
	2.	
	3.	
	4.	
	5.	
2.	1.	
	2.	
	3.	
	4.	
	5.	
3.	1.	
	2.	
	3.	
	4.	
	5.	
4.	1.	
	2.	
	3.	
	4.	
	5.	
5.	1.	
	2.	
	3.	
	4.	
	5.	

CHAPTER 4

Understanding the Stigma of Progressive Memory Loss: Managing Your Responses to the Behaviors of Others

What is stigma and why is it a concern for people with memory loss? At first, the importance of talking about stigma may not be clear to you. Some may not experience stigma, while others may meet people each day with a stigmatized view of those with memory loss. Stigma is a negative view or perception that is common in society about others with a particular illness or disease. Illnesses that cause impaired thinking and mental ability, including memory loss, often result in stigma. Stigma and the negative views that go along with it can cause negative responses in those around you. These responses are caused by false beliefs about people with progressive memory loss and other illnesses. Almost any illness that affects how one thinks or behaves will cause some negative responses or false beliefs. These false beliefs result in a stigmatized view of the individual. These false beliefs can cause others to respond with hurtful, inappropriate comments or reactions to those with memory loss.

Society may encourage this stigmatized view of the person with memory loss by how the person is portrayed or talked about in public. How can someone with memory loss change society's response to them? Changing society's response may be out of your control. However, you can change how *you* respond to the negative reactions and behaviors of people around you. In this chapter, we will describe ways to manage your responses to stigma, giving you the help you need to keep stigma from affecting you in a negative way.

People who have a stigmatizing illness, such as Alzheimer's disease and other forms of progressive memory loss, often react in a personal way to the stigmatizing behaviors of others. This response is called "person stigma." The person stigma experienced by people with memory loss can result in lower self-esteem, lower sense of competency, and a decrease in ability to function. As you can see, the effects of stigma are so negative that they can cause you to withdraw from activities and lower your overall quality of life. So, learning how to change your responses to the negative behaviors of others may improve your quality of life and how you adapt to the memory loss.

Why stigma happens

Why are illnesses like Alzheimer's disease, dementia, or other causes of progressive memory loss stigmatized illnesses? Several features of illnesses that cause memory loss may result in a stigmatized response by others. First, people with memory loss have some difficulty with their thinking and their mental ability. The individual may be viewed as having an impaired mind. This view by others is one reason why those with memory loss are often "talked over" or about in public as if they were not there. Because of the memory loss, people often assume that you are unable to understand what is being said and that you are not able to respond appropriately. Although you know this is not true, you may be placed in the position of being talked about or over without having any control over the situation. This behavior by others is very negative and unnecessary. Unfortunately, this behavior occurs often in our society and can result in a negative experience for you.

Another reason that people around you may respond in a stigmatizing way is the discomfort they feel about the cause of the memory loss. Older people often think that "this could be me." Older adults may fear that in a few years they could be facing the same challenges and concerns as you. This fear and concern for their own wellbeing can make others uncomfortable in your presence. This discomfort in others is not something you cause directly or can even control. Sadly, however, this discomfort in others can cause them to respond negatively to you. Valued friendships can be lost because a friend or co-worker is just too uncomfortable about their own future to be a friend to you. In addition to their own discomfort, others are also not sure how you will respond to them. They know you have some difficulty with memory and thinking, so they are never quite sure what to say or how to approach you. They are not sure you will understand them or that you will respond to them as you have in the past. Again, many of these fears and concerns are not accurate or based on reality. However, these fears in others affect how they will respond to you.

One illness that is a common cause of progressive memory loss is Alzheimer's disease. In fact, many people believe that everyone who has memory loss has Alzheimer's disease. Many illnesses can cause memory loss, but Alzheimer's disease just happens to be the most common one. Alzheimer's disease can be connected to an error or fault in a gene or chromosome, making this illness even more stigmatizing. Any disease that can be carried within a family through a gene that is passed from one person to another can result in stigma. Because the disease is passed from one person to another in a family, others outside the family fear that they could catch the disease by just being with you. Although this belief is totally wrong, it does cause others to respond to individuals with Alzheimer's disease in a negative or hurtful way.

Alzheimer's disease and other types of progressive memory loss also occur mostly in older adults. Just being older may cause others to expect less of you. Even without memory loss, older adults are often viewed as being less able. This view encourages negative responses by others. This negative view by others also limits the extent to which older adults can function at their highest level in society. As others view you as older and less able, they expect less of you and provide fewer chances for you to do the things you are still capable of doing. All of these reasons cause others to react with stigmatizing behaviors to those with progressive memory loss.

The picture is not all negative—thankfully! Some events have happened in the last few years that have affected the stigma of memory loss positively. Some very famous people such as President Ronald Reagan have made public their diagnosis of Alzheimer's disease. This public announcement has allowed the disease to be talked about more openly. Also, making an accurate diagnosis of Alzheimer's disease and other causes of memory loss has decreased some of the mystery about these illnesses. Treatments for progressive memory loss have also increased in the last few years. The increase in positive treatments has allowed memory loss and Alzheimer's disease to be seen as being treatable and it is hoped that some day they will be curable. All of these positive events have begun a movement toward decreases in stigma by the public and society at large. However, people with memory loss still encounter negative responses from others at a personal level. These negative encounters are caused by the stigmatized behaviors of others. Persons with memory loss in the support groups that I have led still often talk about the things that their friends or co-workers have said to them that have been very hurtful. So, while the stigma of memory loss may be declining in the general public, on a personal level, individuals with memory loss are still affected by stigma.

People with memory loss do not always know how to respond to the negative behaviors resulting from stigma. They often cannot stop the negative responses of others from affecting how they feel about themselves. The stories on the following two pages are true examples of a positive and negative response to the stigma of progressive memory loss.

Anne's story

A younger woman in her late fifties, Anne was a member of our support group for people with memory loss. Anne had worked until just a few years before joining the support group. Because of her young age, Anne did not qualify for many retirement benefits, and work had been an important part of her life before her diagnosis. As work was important to her, Anne continued to go back to the workplace and eat lunch with her co-workers at least once a week. After one lunch, as Anne was leaving the cafeteria, another co-worker who Anne had not seen for some time walked up to her. The person stopped and looked at Anne in amazement. The co-worker then went on to say, "What are you doing here? I thought you were too sick to be at work! I thought they had put you in a home!" You can imagine how hard this was for Anne to hear. She had never thought that an old friend would say such a hurtful thing. To Anne and her friends, Anne still belonged "at work." As Anne's friends enjoyed being with her, they assumed others would see their lunches together as being positive for everyone.

Anne talked about this negative response from an old friend at the next support group meeting. As usual, the members of the support group offered Anne advice and encouragement. Many of the suggestions on how to respond to such a negative incident involved using humor. One group member suggested that next time this happened that Anne say, "Yes, I just got out of the home for today, but I have go back tonight." Most group members suggested that Anne tried not to let the remark hurt her and not to take it too seriously. The group members believed that using humor as a response would show Anne's co-worker how inappropriate and hurtful his remark was. Anne took the advice of the group and continued to meet her friends for lunch every week. Anne decided to use humor as one response if a hurtful comment or meeting happened again.

The important parts of this true story of a stigmatizing behavior from others are the ways in which Anne learned to deal with stigma. Anne did not let this very negative meeting change how she thought about herself. Although she was upset about what happened, she did not think less of herself. She understood that her co-worker was wrong in his beliefs about her and her illness. She also understood that she could do something to help herself if this negative response happened again. After this experience of stigma, Anne continued in many different activities outside her home. Because of the support and encouragement of the group,

Anne was able to learn how to deal with these types of responses and not let them affect her in a negative way.

The second story describes what can happen when a person with memory loss does not know how to respond to stigma.

Helen's story

Helen was in her seventies when she was diagnosed with Alzheimer's disease. Helen would go to church every Sunday even though she did not always remember everyone's name and sometimes had a hard time following the sermon. Church had always been important to Helen and it was a big part of her life. She enjoyed going to church with her husband. She could also remember all the words to her favorite hymns. So, going to church was a positive activity for Helen. One Sunday, another member of the church greeted Helen and said, "I didn't know you were still coming to church. What are you doing here?" This remark both alarmed Helen and hurt her feelings. She had never thought of herself as not *belonging* in church. However, the remark from this church member made Helen feel as if she no longer should be coming to church. She really did not know how to respond to this unkind remark.

After this comment, Helen refused to go to church even though her husband wanted her to go with him. She eventually stopped many of her other social activities. She was very careful about where she went and who she would be seeing when she did go out. She finally limited her activities away from home only to events that included family members. Sadly, Helen limited her social activities much more than she needed to, as she still enjoyed being with others. As she became more withdrawn, she also became depressed. Without outside support and help to manage these difficult situations, Helen was not able to deal with her negative encounter in a positive way. In the end, Helen also had more difficulty managing the effects of her memory loss. Helen's negative outcome could have been prevented if she would have had some help to deal with the negative and thoughtless behaviors of others.

Effects of stigma on people with memory loss

Would you know if you were being treated in a different or negative way as a result of the stigma of memory loss? Would you be able to recognize the effects of stigma on your life? People with memory loss experience stigma in many different ways. However, the responses to stigma are similar. One common result of stigma is that you and others may place unneeded limits on your activities. You may decide to give up activities because of fears of negative responses from and behaviors of others. Family members may want to protect you—or themselves—from stigma and may place limits on your activities as well. One of the biggest mistakes I have seen family members make is taking away "too much too soon." So your activities may become more limited, both by you and your family, to protect you from stigma and the negative responses of others.

Stigma is often seen when deception is used with people with memory loss. It is not uncommon for others to distort the truth when talking with you about concerns or issues. For example, a family member might tell you that no funds are left in a bank account for fear that you might spend the money without their knowing it. The money might actually still be available, but the family member might think it is in your best interest to not know the money is still there. Tricks or open deception might also be used. A family member might tell you that you are going to one place, and then take you to a different location—somewhere you might have said you did not want to go. Family members and others generally do not see these as being negative actions. They often feel as if they are acting in your best interests or that they are protecting you. However, these deceptive actions generally have the reverse effect. They often, instead, create in you a sense of not trusting others. By using deception, your rights as a person and your needs are being denied. The use of deception is one behavior that stigma produces in others. This result of stigma can cause future problems as your trust in others declines. This loss of trust may make you feel more alone or misunderstood.

Other responses that are typical of the stigma of memory loss are ignoring behaviors of others. Friends, family members, and even healthcare providers may treat you as if you are just not there. People often will talk over you or talk about you when you are present as if you do not understand or cannot respond to what is being said. One woman I knew well, Sara, lived with her daughter. When I visited Sara, her daughter would talk openly in front of her about how stressful it was to have her mother in the home. Sara knew and understood exactly what her daughter was saying. Over several months, Sara became more and more depressed. When I talked with Sara, she would tell me how her daughter's words were hurtful and how they made her feel sad and depressed. Even when I explained this to the daughter, she would not change her behavior or see the need to watch what was said in Sara's presence. The daughter was totally unaware of Sara's increasing depression. She was also unaware that her comments were part of the cause of Sara's depression. The daughter's stigmatized view of her mother prevented her from knowing that Sara understood her words and took in what was being said about her. It may seem to you that this type of behavior from a family member is not common or likely to happen to you. However, this ignoring response is very common, even from family members. These ignoring behaviors of others are associated with the stigma of progressive memory loss.

When a person with memory loss is treated negatively due to stigma, the needs and wishes of others may override your needs or desires. Thomas Kitwood (1997a, 1997b) talks about how others have a tendency to impose their wishes on individuals with memory loss when they have a stigmatized view of that person. When this happens and your needs are not recognized, others may make choices that would not necessarily be your choices. The stigma of memory loss results in others limiting your voice in decisions about your life. Another stigmatizing response from others can result in others blaming you for changes in your ability. I cannot tell you how often I have heard family members say, "I know he or she can do this if they only tried hard enough." This response from family members may not seem like blaming, but it implies that somehow you can control your ability to carry out a task or previous role. "If only they would try hard enough" implies that you just may not be doing your best to do what others expect of you. I have found it difficult to convince family members that usually you are doing the best you can. The stigma of memory loss interferes with the ability of family members to understand and accept that you may have no direct control over the effects of the memory loss on your behavior or abilities.

You may also encounter stigma from the professionals who provide your healthcare. It is expected that healthcare providers understand the causes of memory loss and do not view the person with memory loss in a stigmatized way. Healthcare providers can be any professional person you see for health-related care, such as physicians, nurse practitioners, physicians' assistants, social workers, and therapists. Even though healthcare providers are professional, their responses to you may be affected by their beliefs about memory loss or older adults in general. You may find that when you see your healthcare provider you may not be asked questions directly about your health or symptoms you are having. Healthcare providers may, instead, direct their questions to your family member or spouse. They may assume that you are not a reliable source of information as you have been diagnosed with an illness that causes memory loss and impaired thinking. Often, healthcare providers are unaware of the fact that early in any illness that causes memory loss you may be a very good source of information.

Another factor that can affect the responses of healthcare providers is how they view your quality of life. Because you are diagnosed with a progressive illness, healthcare professionals often think that your quality of life is lower than it actually is. You are the best expert on your quality of life. However, you may not even be asked about your quality of life. This judgment on the part of healthcare professionals about your quality of life can result in lack of effective treatment for even common illnesses such as high blood pressure or heart disease. If healthcare providers view your future quality of life as being less than it might be, they may not feel it is necessary to provide you with the most effective treatments. These decisions by healthcare professionals can negatively affect your health and your ability to manage other illnesses.

These possible stigmatized responses from healthcare professionals make it necessary for you to be more assertive. You may need to ask your healthcare provider about the most effective treatments for any illness you have. You may need to be more assertive in making sure the healthcare provider understands your wishes about treatment choices. When the healthcare provider asks questions about your health problems, you may find it necessary to make sure your answers are heard, along with the answers given by your family members or spouse. In the early stages of progressive memory loss, especially, the information you provide is valuable for your healthcare provider to hear. You may not be able to change the perceptions of your healthcare provider about your ability. Understanding why your healthcare provider may overlook your views and voice may help you prepare to make sure your wishes are heard. By asserting yourself, you can make sure you are part of the treatment decisions that may affect your health.

On a larger level, we see public advertisements, jokes in the media, and television programs that mock the person with progressive memory loss. Often jokes about memory loss are made at your expense. Just like the common jokes about different ethnic groups, there are jokes about forgetting. Alzheimer's disease is often called "old timer's" disease in a very joking or demeaning way. These jokes are actually making fun about an illness that is completely beyond your control. Also, this type of mocking can increase the stigmatized views of others. These negative messages can hurt your self-esteem. Public mocking or joking can increase the feeling of being set apart from other people. Studies are attempting to find ways to fight this type of public mocking of people with progressive memory loss. Until these studies are completed, the reality is that you may be affected by some of these public negative views.

To help fight the effects of stigma, you, your family members and healthcare providers can learn about why stigma happens and why others respond to you the way they do. This knowledge will help you to use your abilities, resources, and support systems to help you decrease the effects of stigma. For you, managing or decreasing the effects of stigma can help you stay active and maintain your self-esteem. To assist you, the next section describes some actions and interventions that may help you manage the effects of stigma.

Interventions to help manage stigma

Support groups

In Chapter 1, we described support groups as being helpful when accepting the diagnosis of progressive memory loss. Support groups may also be helpful in managing the effects of stigma. Group members share their experiences and successes, and they can offer suggestions on ways to manage the negative behaviors of others that result from stigma. This allows you to not only learn from others what works best, but you can also compare your own situation with those of the other group members. Often, people with progressive memory loss feel as if they are alone. You might feel as if no one understands you. The stigmatizing behaviors of others reinforce this view. Being part of a support group helps you know that others understand what you are facing and know that others share your experiences. Being part of a support group and having positive responses from others also results in a decrease in your own negative thoughts. You can have hope when you see other people with memory loss managing the negative responses caused by stigma.

Behavioral therapies

The second intervention to help manage stigma is part of the cognitive and behavioral therapy introduced in Chapter 1. Behavioral therapy focuses on positive beliefs about yourself. Behavioral therapies are designed to give you ways to cope with the negative responses of others. In behavioral therapies, your negative views of yourself are presented in a more realistic way to reduce the distortions or false mental pictures that you have of yourself. The therapies give you positive or more accurate thoughts to replace the negative thoughts. Also, behavioral therapies help you have a sense of control over your moods and your life. These more positive views and increased sense of control help you respond more positively to the stigmatizing behaviors of others.

In working with people with memory loss, I have found that many individuals with memory loss see themselves negatively mostly because of the responses of others. Even people who functioned in high-level positions, such as lawyers and physicians, would describe themselves using words such as "useless" or "stupid." These negative statements tell us that individuals with memory loss identify too strongly with their illness and the negative behaviors of others. The mental exercises used in behavioral therapies help you to correct these negative self-beliefs and responses. The therapies also help you to focus more on your abilities, rather than losses. Those with memory loss are taught to use and trust their own behaviors and abilities. They are also shown how to use positive behaviors to respond to the negative behaviors of others. Behavioral therapies help you prepare for negative responses of others in social interactions. Responses to negative behaviors of others are often rehearsed in the therapies so that you are more prepared to respond positively when an encounter happens. Behavioral therapies and support groups can help you find positive ways to keep the negative responses of others from damaging your self-esteem and quality of life. Your healthcare provider can assist you in finding a professional who provides behavioral therapy. This person is often a social worker licensed in individual and family therapy or a mental health professional with experience in behavioral therapy.

Normalization

Another way to manage stigma is to use what is referred to as normalization. Normalization is a process of attempting to keep your life in balance or as normal as possible following your diagnosis. One response to the stigmatizing behaviors of others is to withdraw from your usual activities. This change in your level of activities can then cause a sense of loss of what has been normal in your life before. Your spouse and other family members can also feel this change from normal, as it might affect their daily routines as well. So, trying to normalize your daily activities and routines is one way to keep positive patterns that are consistent with your past.

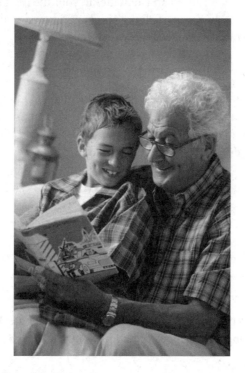

Keeping normal activity patterns in your life can be made easier by setting yourself up for a positive response in social activities. You can design social activities for success. An example of this might be something as simple as eating a meal away from home. Dining out with a large group of people might cause you to become confused or not be able to follow a conversation. However, if you dine out with a small group, perhaps no more than two to four other people, this small group allows you to talk with others more easily without fear of embarrassment. Also, you can use little reminders before dining out, such as writing down the names of the people who will be at the dinner on a slip of paper and keeping the paper close at hand. If you forget someone's name, then you can just look at the paper to remind yourself of their name. These little ways of protecting yourself in social activities can result in fewer stigmatizing behaviors from others as they see you in a normal situation.

To normalize your life as much as possible, you may want to think about what makes your day normal or routine. In other words, you can identify what is an important part of your day-to-day activities. Once you identify what these activities are, you can find ways to adapt them to make them safe and successful for you. You may then feel comfortable continuing these activities. Keeping activities from the past in your life provides you with a greater sense of normalcy. Although this may seem like a very simple intervention, just finding ways to keep the same pattern and activities in your life can be very helpful in staying active, without fear of failing. The more normal your life is, the less likely others are to treat you in a stigmatized way.

Humor

It has often been said that laughter is a good medicine. This applies to managing the negative behaviors of others as well. One of the most successful ways to respond to a negative behavior from another person is a humorous or light response. If you do not take the other person's behavior seriously, they may begin to question their own behavior. Laughing off a negative remark also helps make it seem less serious or hurtful to you. If you can laugh at someone else's mistakes, as well as your own, then it is less likely that you will take in the response and let it affect your self-esteem and self-confidence. Members of our support group describe using humor more often than any other response to hurtful or negative comments from others.

Are you ready?

Managing stigma can make a difference in your quality of life. While you might not be able to change another person's impressions of you, you can change how you respond to others. By not taking in or believing the negative responses from others, you will be more positive about yourself and your abilities. Using the positive interventions suggested in this chapter can help you to have more positive relationships with others. Much of your self-image and your thoughts about yourself are formed through your interactions with others. So, increasing positive ways to interact with others will help you keep a positive image of yourself. These positive interactions will result in better long-term relationships with the people who are part of your social network and support system. By limiting the effect that stigma has on your life, you can help life remain as normal as possible for everyone, including your family and friends. The positive effects of managing stigma will help you limit the extent to which memory loss directly affects your life. At the end of this chapter you will find a list of positive actions you can take to help manage the stigma you experience. You may find it helpful to review this list when others treat you in a stigmatizing way. These positive actions may help prevent stigma from having a negative effect on your life.

STEPS TO MANAGE STIGMA

- Join a support group: group members offer suggestions on ways to manage the negative behaviors of others.

- Use behavioral therapy to help you focus on positive beliefs about yourself.

- Find positive ways to cope with the negative responses of others.

- Use mental exercises to help you correct negative self-beliefs and responses.

- Focus on your abilities, rather than losses.

- Keep your life in balance or as normal as possible after your diagnosis.

- Keep daily activities and routines as consistent as possible with your past.

- Design social activities to be successful.

- Respond to negative behaviors from another person with humor or a light response.

- Educate others about memory loss to help them understand your abilities and needs as a person.

CHAPTER 5

Communicating with Others

People with progressive memory loss often have difficulty communicating with others. The type and extent of communication difficulties varies from one individual to another. As memory loss progresses, communication may become even more difficult. This chapter will focus on:

1. the importance of maintaining communication

2. types of communication issues for people with progressive memory loss and their conversation partners

3. strategies that you and your conversation partners can use to improve communication.

In this chapter, the term "conversation partners" will be used. Conversation partners are usually people who are close to you. For example, your conversation partners could be your spouse, other family members, and friends. The term "partners" is part of conversation, as it is important to realize that no one communicates alone. When discussing communication, it would be easy to blame any communication problems on the person with progressive memory loss. However, communication is always a two-way process. A speaker and a listener are always part of the conversation. Both conversation partners are responsible for good communication.

You have probably heard the expression: "It takes two to tango." Well, it also takes at least two to communicate. Think about communication as being like dancing. We go back and forth with words. It would be difficult for one person to dance without a partner. And even though most of us are not perfect dancers, or communicators, we still enjoy doing it. If we step on our partner's toes once in awhile, do we give up and quit dancing? No, we keep trying to dance because it is a good way to feel close to another person. Even if our communication is not perfect, we still need to keep communicating. Good communication helps hold people together. For you, a person with progressive memory loss, it is important to keep communicating for as long as possible.

Some of the benefits of communicating with others include:

1. making your wishes known

2. being part of making decisions

3. expressing your emotions

4. relieving loneliness

5. maintaining your identity.

Communicating with others can create or relieve tension, depending on the ability of both individuals to be flexible and understanding. The following stories will give you examples of both positive and negative outcomes of communication.

Nora's story

Nora has progressive memory loss. Nora and her husband, Michael, have been married for over 50 years. Nora and Michael are both retired and spend most of their day together. The have always enjoyed talking to one another. With Nora's memory loss, she might lose track of the topic of the conversation. At times, Nora may start talking about a completely new topic. Sometimes Michael helps her get back to the original topic. Other times, though, Michael enjoys talking about the new topic with Nora. Nora sometimes repeats herself. Michael doesn't mind the repetition. Nora's favorite words to Michael are, "I love you." He says: "She can repeat it as often as she likes." Both Nora and Michael know that perfect communication is not possible. However, they still enjoy talking to each other as Michael is patient and wants to talk with Nora. As Nora cares very much for Michael, she is willing to try to communicate despite her memory loss. This cooperation between Nora and Michael has allowed them to have positive communication for years after Nora's diagnosis of memory loss.

Hal's story

Soon after being diagnosed with progressive memory loss, Hal began having difficulty talking. When he started to speak, he often could not find the right words to say. Hal had always been shy, so talking with others had never been easy for him. Now that Hal had trouble finding the right words, he was even less comfortable talking with others. Hal began spending more time alone. When Hal's family visited, he would sit in a corner away from others. The less Hal talked, the more difficult his speech became. With fewer contacts with family members and friends, Hal became depressed as his time alone increased. Hal's fear of making mistakes when talking with others led to a faster decline in thinking ability and memory.

Both Nora and Hal had similar levels of memory loss. The main difference in the way they managed their communication problems was their willingness to talk to others. Hal became easily discouraged and stopped trying to communicate. Nora, who had always enjoyed talking, found different ways to communicate her feelings. As communication is needed for relationships, Nora was able to still feel connected to those she loved, while Hal became more and more lonely. The difference in communication alone helped Nora stay active and connected to others.

An important part of good communication is attending to what the other person says. For people with progressive memory loss, it may be more difficult to attend for long periods of time. The following suggestions may help you maintain your attention during a conversation.

1. Remove distractions from the area where you will have the conversation. Turn off the radio and television. Talk where you cannot hear other conversations.

2. Look directly at the other person while you are talking and listening.

3. Do not try to do anything else while you are talking and listening.

4. Do not have long or complicated discussions when you are tired. Try having more conversations in the morning when you are feeling well rested.

5. If a long or complicated discussion is required, try breaking the conversation into smaller pieces. For example, when planning for a vacation, you do not need to discuss everything at the same time. One day, you could discuss where to go on vacation. The next day, you could discuss the travel arrangements. The following day, you could discuss lodging.

Perceptions of others

Your most frequent conversation partners are likely to be your spouse, other family members, and close friends. These people care about you and may feel protective of you. Because of these protective feelings, they may engage in what is called "overaccommodation." Overaccommodation in communication may occur when people talk down to you because you have memory loss. Sometimes overaccommodation sounds like baby talk. Overaccommodation may also occur when your conversation partners try to protect you from certain types of information. If your conversation partners talk down to you, you could lose confidence in your own communication abilities. You could become discouraged and stop trying to communicate. If you feel that your conversation partners are too overaccommodating, you might try making statements like these:

1. "Please talk to me as an adult."

2. "Please listen to what I have to say."

3. "Please tell me the truth."

"Underaccommodation" in communication may occur when people talk too rapidly or too softly and do not consider your individual communication needs. If your conversation partners are too underaccommodating, you might become frustrated by not being able to keep up with the conversation. You could become discouraged and stop trying to communicate. If you feel that your conversation partners are too underaccommodating, you might try making statements like these:

1. "Please slow down a little."

2. "Please repeat that for me."

3. "Please explain that to me."

Finding the right amount of accommodation or adjustment in communication is an individual process. For example, for some people, this book may seem too easy or overaccommodating. For others, this book may seem too difficult or underaccommodating. We tried to write this book for a wide audience. In individual conversations, however, it is easier to adjust communication to the appropriate level. Both overaccommodation and underaccommodation in communication could affect you negatively.

Richard's story

Richard has progressive memory loss. Before he retired, Richard owned a large business. His wife died the year before he was diagnosed with. He now lives in a residence for older adults with memory loss. He hates the way the nursing assistants talk to him. "They talk to me in that high-pitched, sing-song voice, just like I'm a baby. I am *not* a baby. And don't call me honey or sweetie either. My name is Richard or Mr. Smith."

The nursing assistants were using overaccommodation in communication. Overaccommodation may cause anger and frustration for the person with memory loss. In this story, Richard needed to let the nursing assistants know how he felt about their communication. The nursing assistants, like family members, needed to learn how to communicate in an appropriate and respectful way with someone with memory loss.

Common communication errors

When communication errors occur, what happens? Typically, when a communication error occurs, one or both partners complete a "conversational repair." Something in the conversation "broke down" and is then repaired by the speaker or listener or both. These conversational repairs take place all the time in everyday conversations. It is not just people with progressive memory loss who make conversational errors. We all make conversational errors. These errors are usually small and are easily repaired. Here are some examples of the types of conversational errors and repairs that are fairly common. In these examples, Mary is the person with memory loss and Harold is her husband and conversation partner.

1. Mary says: "My brother lives in London" and then says: "Oh, no, I mean he lives in New York now." Mary noticed and corrected her own error. Harold does not need to say anything about the minor error.

2. Mary says: "I like that animal at the zoo." Harold might ask: "What animal?" This is a clarification question. Mary then might say: "I mean the chimpanzee." So Mary added a clarification for Harold. In this case, Mary could say the exact word that she meant.

3. Mary says: "I like that movie." Harold might ask: "What movie?"
    Again, this is a clarification question. But Mary might not be able
    to say the name of the movie. This issue is often referred to as
    word-finding difficulty. Mary might say: "That movie where the
    children go through the wardrobe." Then Harold might say, "Oh,
    yes, the *Chronicles of Narnia*." So even though Mary couldn't think
    of the name of the movie, she was still able to give enough
    information so that Harold would know what she was talking
    about. Mary used a communication strategy called "talking around
    the word" or circumlocution. This communication technique is
    important for people with progressive memory loss. Don't give up
    trying to communicate just because you cannot think of the exact
    word. Often, if you can talk about what you mean, your
    conversation partner will know the exact word and say it.

4. Harold says: "Let's go to that restaurant…you know, that one you
    like." Mary answers: "Oh, yes the place with Indian food." Harold
    says: "Oh, yes, that one." In this example, neither Harold nor Mary
    can remember the exact name of the restaurant but they both know
    which restaurant they are talking about. Even though Harold does
    not have progressive memory loss, he too, like most people, has
    times when he cannot think of the exact word that he wants to use.

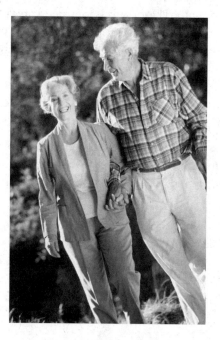

What all the above examples have in common is that both conversation partners were patient and kept trying to communicate until they understood each other. Do you see now that conversational errors and repairs occur often in our everyday communication? Researchers like Orange and Lubinski (1996) have studied conversational errors and repairs. The good news is that among individuals with mild memory loss and their partners, about three-quarters (75%) of conversations were free of errors. Even among people with more memory loss and their partners, about two-thirds (64%) of conversations were free of errors. So, most of the time, people with progressive memory loss can and do communicate successfully with their conversation partners. Even when conversation errors do occur, most of these errors can be easily repaired.

Most conversational errors are very minor and do not need to be repaired or pointed out. If you have a conversation partner who constantly notices and repairs your errors, this can be very distracting and discouraging. You might try making statements like these:

1. "If you notice that I have made a major error, please gently repair the error."

2. "If I make a minor error, please just ignore it. I will ignore your minor errors. We all make mistakes."

3. "If I ask you to help me repair an error, please do so in an understanding way. Please do not embarrass me by saying things like: 'Don't you know that?' 'Can't you remember that?'"

Anne's story

Anne had progressive memory loss. She lived with her adult daughter, Beth. Whenever Anne made mistake in a conversation, Beth always noticed and corrected her. Most of Anne's mistakes were very small and did not need to be corrected. Beth mistakenly thought that correcting her mother regularly would improve her mother's speech. Instead, the constant interruptions and corrections made Anne feel even more nervous about talking. After a few months, Anne stopped talking much at all. She became socially isolated and depressed. Her ability to function independently rapidly declined. Beth placed her mother in a nursing home because she could no longer talk or take care of herself.

In the above story, a family member concentrated too much on trying to make sure that conversations were perfect. It would have been better for the daughter to have regular, nonjudgmental conversations with her mother.

Ways to improve communication

Edwards and Chapman (2004a, 2004b) studied family members and their communication styles. They found that the most satisfying and effective communication style was equal participation by the communication partners. In this style of communication, both conversation partners are recognized as equal partners. One partner is not considered more important or more correct. This style, however, recognizes that two conversation partners may have different strengths and weaknesses. Good communication will take these differences into account. Conversation partners can talk about and share decisions. To continue to communicate as well as possible for as long as possible, you and your conversation partners must practice good communication on a regular basis. For people with progressive memory loss, communication takes more time and effort. Sometimes you may feel as if it's just not worth it. If you get frustrated and quit trying to communicate, your communication skills will worsen. Good communication is a skill. You must practice regularly.

Lucy's story on the next page is an example of positive communication practice. Here are some communication activities for you and your conversation partners to practice:

1. Take turns choosing conversation topics.

2. Take turns starting a conversation.

3. Take turns listening and talking.

4. Take turns asking for help or clarification during a conversation.

5. Take turns giving help or clarification during a conversation.

6. Take turns talking about your feelings.

Many lists of do's and don'ts have been written for communicating with people who have memory loss. For example, organizations like the Alzheimer's Association have lists that suggest communication strategies. Some of these lists are not as helpful as they could be, however. First of all, the list usually focuses on what the family member should do. The family member is only half of the communication partnership. In this chapter, I have tried to add what the person with memory loss can do for him or herself to make communication better. To improve communication, both conversation partners need help. The other

---

Lucy's story

Lucy has progressive memory loss. She lives with her sister, Velma. Lucy and Velma have made a game out of practicing conversations. Velma has a large jar with slips of paper in it. On each slip of paper, a topic is listed. When Lucy and Velma talk, if neither one can think of a topic, they draw a slip of paper. Velma cuts the topics out of the newspaper so they both laugh and say, "We never know what we will be talking about next." One day, their topic was about some newly discovered dinosaur bones. Both of them had trouble talking about the dinosaur bones and finally turned to a different topic. During their conversations, Velma uses a timer so that each one of them will have the same amount of time to talk and to listen. Lucy and Velma are enjoying themselves when they talk together. They have invented some ways to keep their conversations fun and interesting. They both realize that the actual topic of conversation is not nearly as important as the closeness they feel while they are talking and laughing.

---

problem with these lists of do's and don'ts is that some of the strategies are not really helpful. Because the strategies have been repeated so many times, many people believe they are helpful even though some of them are not. Some researchers like Jeff Small and others (Small *et al.*, 2003) have studied which strategies tend to improve communication for individuals with memory loss. The strategies listed below have been shown to *improve* communication for those with memory loss.

1. Remove distractions from the area of the conversation. For example, turn off the radio or television.

2. Use shorter sentences. Shorter sentences allow people with memory loss to follow the thought of the sentence. For example, shorter sentences have been used in this book to help you understand each point.

3. Ask only "yes" or "no" questions. Because this strategy is somewhat controversial, it is discussed in more detail below.

It is true that when a conversation partner asks only yes or no questions, the person with memory loss will be more successful in answering. It is easier for a person with memory loss to say only yes or no than to have to say a complete sentence. However, even though this is easier, it may not be better. Asking only yes or no questions may be a form of overaccommodation.

Overaccommodation occurs when your conversation partner talks down to you. Then you do not have a chance to practice your communication. Also, if your conversation partners only ask you yes or no questions, they may not even be asking you the right questions. For example, your conversation partner could ask you, "Do you want to go to the movie?" If you say "Yes", that is fine, and you will both go to a movie. But what if you say "No"? How will your partner know what you want? Many times, asking only yes or no questions may not be the best way to communicate. It might be better for your conversation partner to ask you something like: "What would you like to do today?" Then the two of you can have a conversation about what to do. This is the mutual participation style of communication. Using yes or no questions may work well in some situations. However, I do not recommend using only yes or no questions.

Your conversation partner, usually a family member, may quiz you or test you during a conversation. Family members often, by mistake, think this is a good way to help you with your memory. Your conversation partner may say something like, "Now, tell me the name of our friend who is going to visit later." Most of the time, this type of quizzing makes you feel embarrassed and defeated. Quizzing is also not appropriate as part of conversation. If your conversation partner wants to help you with your memory, then a time should be set aside just to work on memory or word-finding skills—if that is something you want to work on as well. If your conversation partner starts to quiz you during a conversation, you might need to say something like, "Please don't try to test my memory when we are talking. My doctors test my memory for me." This simple statement might help your conversation partner know that it is not appropriate for them to quiz you. Your conversation partner should help with your memory only if you ask for help. Quizzing someone during conversation is never appropriate. Your embarrassment may make you more hesitant to talk when others are around.

One communication strategy that is often recommended is for the conversation partner to speak slowly to the person with progressive memory loss. This strategy is *not* usually helpful. Speaking too fast can be confusing for anyone. Speaking more slowly than normal, however, does not improve communication. It may be that slow speech seems too abnormal to be understood. Also, people with memory loss may have trouble remembering and understanding a complete sentence if it is stated too slowly. The best strategy is to speak at a normal pace. Conversation should be "not to fast" and "not too slow" but "just right."

Another communication strategy that is often suggested is for the conversation partners to repeat sentences as necessary. Everyone agrees that repeating sentences is sometimes necessary. The controversy is about *how* the sentence should be repeated. Some experts say that the sentence should be repeated exactly as it was originally stated. For example, the conversation partner might say: "Let's go to the holiday ceremony at the church tonight." If the person with memory loss does not completely understand the statement, the conversation partner could keep repeating the sentence exactly as originally stated (verbatim). The reason for repeating the exact same sentence is to try to avoid adding more words and confusion. On the other hand, the conversation partner could change the wording a little (paraphrase). The new sentence could be something like: "Let's go to church tonight to celebrate Christmas." The reason for using slightly different words is that the new sentence may be better understood. No clear evidence exists that one of these strategies is better than the other. In other words, when repeating sentences, one or both strategies can be used. You and your conversation partner may want to practice using both of these strategies. With practice, you may know which strategy works best for you to help understand what your conversation partner is saying.

Communicating with outsiders

So far, this chapter has focussed on how you can improve communication with your regular conversation partners, usually family or friends. Sometimes, though, you may need to communicate with people you do not know. For example, you may meet strangers at a shop or the library, or at a restaurant. Strangers are not likely to know anything at all about progressive memory loss. Strangers may have little or no patience with your special communication needs. They may say or do things that hurt your feelings or make you angry. Unfortunately, you cannot change the behavior of others. It is important, however, that you not take these negative communication experiences personally. When you know that you are going to be around strangers, you may want to take one of your regular conversation partners with you. Your partner should not take over the conversation, however. Think of your partner as the person who will help out if the communication becomes too difficult for you. Continuing to interact with others in the real world is an important part of your communication practice.

Another communication situation that you will encounter is the visit with a healthcare provider. This type of communication usually involves a "triad" or three people: your healthcare provider, you, and usually one of your family members. A close family member or friend should go with you to all healthcare provider visits. The family member or friend can be of great help to you before, during, and after the visit. However, the main problem with having three people at the visit is that now three people are trying to communicate. Throughout this chapter, you have seen how difficult communication can be for even two people. With three people, or a triad, communication becomes even more difficult. A typical communication problem with triads is this: the healthcare provider may begin talking to your family member or friend and completely ignore you. Although healthcare providers have years of specialized education, very few of them have been trained to communicate with people with progressive memory loss. In fact, after reading this chapter, you probably know more about communication than many of your healthcare providers. Adams and Gardiner (2005) wrote an article about communication in triads. Some of their ideas about how to communicate in triads at a healthcare provider visit include the following.

1. Ask for distractions to be removed from the room.

2. Ideally, the seating should be arranged like a triangle. Each person should be about the same distance from each other. Each person should be able to see and talk to the other two people.

3. You may need to raise your hand or interrupt the conversation to get the attention of the healthcare provider. It may seem rude to interrupt; but if you do not, you may not get your turn to talk.

4. Speak up for yourself. You may have to say something like: "Could you please talk to me?" or "I can tell you about my health problem better than anyone."

The healthcare provider and your family member should do the following.

1. Take turns talking and listening.

2. Give you time to answer their questions.

3. Invite you to ask questions.

4. Help you make important decisions.

The healthcare provider and your family member should *not*

1. interrupt you.

2. speak for you; you may need to say: "I'd like to speak for myself."

3. use complex terms and language; you may need to say: "Please explain what you mean by that."

4. talk about you in front of you; you may need to say: "I'm right here. Please talk *to* me not *about* me."

5. have a meeting or conversation in another room without you. This is a form of overprotective communication; you may need to say: "I'd like to know the truth about my health."

Most healthcare providers want to care for you in the best way possible. However, you and your partner may need to help educate the healthcare provider about how to communicate with you. Once your healthcare provider understands what is most helpful, the visits will be easier. You will also feel as if you have more control over your healthcare and decisions about your health.

Other types of communication

Not all communication is verbal or spoken. Some communication is nonverbal. An example of nonverbal communication is touch. Sometimes just holding hands with someone you care about can be better than having a conversation with words, as Jeff's story shows. Nonverbal communication like holding hands and hugging is a good way to express emotions that may be too difficult to talk about.

Jeff's story

One young man, Jeff, was in his early fifties and had been married for only a few years when he was diagnosed with Alzheimer's disease. Jeff loss his ability to use words correctly soon after his diagnosis. As Jeff's memory and thinking declined, he was less and less able to talk. Although Jeff could not talk with his wife, he enjoyed her company and would light up whenever he was with her. Jeff used touch to let his wife know how much he cared. Even though he could not say, I love you, Jeff would look into his wife's eyes, hold her close, and kiss her goodbye whenever she left for work. Jeff's nonverbal expressions of love meant as much to his wife as words. Like Jeff, you can use nonverbal communication to add to your verbal communication. For example, if you are trying to think of the name of a book and can't remember it, you could just pick up the book and show it to your partner. At times, it is easier to let someone know how much you care through touch than through words.

Written information and cues are another type of communication. You may be able to use this type of communication even when you are alone. For example, you might place a note on the front door that reminds you to lock the door when you are leaving the house. You and your partners can place notes around the house to help you function more independently. Using written reminders is often more acceptable than having someone remind you what to do. You can read the note and complete the activity on your own.

Reminiscence is a particular type of communication that you might want to use with your conversation partners. Often, reminiscence starts without either partner even trying. For example, you might be looking at a scrapbook full of pictures and start talking about the weddings of your children. Reminiscence may be enjoyable for both you and your conversation partners. One of the good things about reminiscence is that this type of conversation relies more on long-term memory. You probably have problems with your short-term memory, such as remembering what you ate for dinner yesterday. But your long-term memory is probably still fairly good. You can talk about events from your past and enjoy having a conversation. If you don't remember particular details about the past, don't worry. You can still enjoy reminiscing without a perfect memory. Memories of repeated events (birthdays, holidays, vacations) tend to be better than memories of single events. This is true for all people, not just for people with memory loss. For example, if you attended the weddings of your four children, you are likely to remember that there was a lot of food, everyone had a good time, the bride looked beautiful, and so on. However, you may confuse some of the minor details of each wedding. Do you really care about that? When reminiscing, try to enjoy the process of talking about past events. You do not need to remember everything to enjoy reminiscing with your conversation partners.

Another form of communication is reading. Reading does not necessarily require a partner. Maintaining your reading ability requires practice. I recommend that you continue to read on a daily basis for as long as you can. At some point, you may have more difficulty reading. You might still enjoy having someone read to you or listening to books on tapes.

Professionals who can help

If you have hearing problems, you should be evaluated by a healthcare provider who specializes in hearing, an audiologist. If you need to wear hearing aids, please do so. To communicate well, you need to hear as well as possible. Another source of help with your communication is a speech or language therapist. Speech therapists are health professionals who have several years of education and experience. A speech therapist can assess your specific communication issues. This chapter has provided general information about communication. A speech therapist, however, can evaluate and treat you as an individual. A speech therapist may be able to develop a special plan for you and your conversation partners to improve your overall communication. Ask your healthcare provider if you can be evaluated by a speech therapist.

The suggestions given in this chapter may make communicating much more positive for you. Try not to get discouraged if a conversation is hard or turns out differently than you had hoped. Almost everyone with memory loss has some trouble finding the right words to say. Some people with memory loss have trouble understanding what others are saying to them. You are not alone in your struggles to communicate well. Remember, however, that communicating is important to positive relationships with others. The effort your put into communicating now will be well worth the benefits of staying close and involved with those you love. The guidelines for communicating at the end of this chapter may be used to remind you of ways to help your communication be positive for everyone.

WAYS TO HELP WITH COMMUNICATION

- Turn off the radio and television.

- Focus only on one thought or idea at a time.

- Look directly at the person while you are talking and listening.

- Don't try to do other things while you are talking and listening.

- Accept that conversations are never perfect.

- Ask for repetition and clarification as needed.

- If you can't think of the word you want to say, "talk around the word." The other person may be able to guess the word you want to say.

- Practice, practice, practice both talking and listening.

- Use other forms of communication to make your needs known, such as touch and written communication.

- Enjoy talking with your friends and family.

- If you are being ignored in a conversation or talked about without being included in the conversation, you may need to let others know how you feel. You may need to say things like:

  ◦ "I'd like to speak for myself."

  ◦ "I'm right here. Please talk to me, not about me."

  ◦ "Please explain to me what you are saying."

CHAPTER 6

Staying Active and Functional

With memory loss or changes in mental ability, you may find yourself faced with finding ways to remain as independent as possible. Being active and independent is especially important for younger people diagnosed with diseases that cause memory loss. Some people are diagnosed in their late forties and early fifties, at a time when they are still working, driving, and managing their own finances. People diagnosed earlier in life may be responsible for others as well, such as children in college or young grandchildren. No matter your age, each of you has been active in some type of lifework, hobbies, social activities, and day-to-day tasks. In other words, you face this diagnosis having lived a life full of activities and responsibilities.

In Chapter 4, we described the effects of stigma on your willingness to continue being active and engaged. Along with the stigma of memory loss, changes in your abilities will influence the degree to which you continue with previous activities. Too often, changes in your mental abilities affect not only how well you recall events, but also your ability to do tasks such as math calculations, actions that require multiple steps, or manage more than one task at a time. These changes may lead to frustration, as you want to continue to function just as you did before the diagnosis. In addition to frustration, you may have a tendency to withdraw and just give up trying to do things. It may be too hard to do the day-to-day tasks that you have done all of your life.

You may also find yourself feeling negative about yourself or blaming yourself when you cannot do the things you were used to doing. One of the men in my support group, Frank, often describes himself as being useless. Frank certainly is not useless. He has a number of abilities that he uses each day. However, Frank becomes frustrated and discouraged because the tasks he did before his diagnosis have become more difficult for him. He tends to let this frustration overwhelm him, causing him to *feel* useless when he can still function well. These changes in ability to perform tasks you have done in the past may also leave you feeling unsure of yourself. And, you may find your confidence in your abilities lessening. This lessening confidence, while expected, may result in you being less willing to continue in past activities and productive roles. Many people with memory loss give up valued activities long before they cannot do them just because they lack the confidence to try even when they are still capable of doing the activity.

Some aspects of your environment may make it difficult for you to perform as you have in the past. We live in an "information age" with new products in computers and technology everyday. Just communicating with others may be harder for you as you constantly need to keep up with the latest technology. To offset these difficulties, special programs have been developed to make using technology easier, including simple instructions to use cell phones. Instead of becoming frustrated and giving up on trying technology, you may need to learn to use new technology through a different method, suited to your abilities.

Our physical world is changing quickly today as well. Most communities are growing and changing. These changes mean there are new roads, shopping areas, and housing developments. These changes also require you to learn new ways of getting around, which can be frustrating and discouraging. Also, as we become more mobile, we are in contact with a lot more people. Years ago, a family might drive for a vacation and meet or talk to very few people. Today, with air and group travel, you are forced to be in close contact with many new people and faces. The increased complexity of your world, including getting around and traveling, makes it much more difficult for you to take in what is going on around you. The more complex your world becomes, the more you are expected to remember. This increased complexity can work against someone with memory loss.

Some of the following stories illustrate different ways to manage your changing memory and abilities to stay active and functioning at your highest level possible. The first story is about a man, Al, who is successful in staying active and involved. The second story describes a woman, Dorothy, who is not as successful in functioning at her highest possible level.

Al's story

Al was a retired professional, who had worked as an engineer. In addition to his work, Al was highly involved in community activities. He had weekly meetings with retired professionals from his work. When Al was diagnosed with Alzheimer's disease, he faced the reality that his driving was affected. This change in his ability to drive could have caused Al to stop doing activities with his professional friends. However, instead of stopping his activities, Al managed his changing abilities in some very creative ways. One of the first things Al did was to arrange for one of his friends to pick him up for his weekly meetings. Al also agreed to take on only those tasks with which he felt comfortable. Al's hobby of growing orchids was fairly complex. Instead of giving up growing orchids, Al just scaled back his collection to make it manageable. Al continued to read the literature from his profession on a weekly basis. This helped him stay in touch with what was going on in his field and allowed him to be more comfortable in his weekly meetings with retired professionals. Al continued to attend church, and with his wife, watched their grandchildren each week. Al's willingness to try different ways to stay active allowed him to continue with most of the activities that he had done previously for years after he was diagnosed with Alzheimer's disease. Al was able to stay happy and outgoing, even as his memory loss increased.

Dorothy's story

Dorothy was an older woman who lived by herself in a rural community when she was diagnosed with progressive memory loss. Because Dorothy was somewhat isolated, driving was the only way for her to get around. When she realized she could no longer drive safely, she began to stop doing many of her usual activities. Dorothy stopped shopping and going to church, and her women's groups. Her withdrawal from activities increased when she became confused on a long trip with a group of church members. Because she became confused on the trip, she decided to stop traveling, even though she had enjoyed traveling with groups for a long time. Dorothy eventually gave up her home and moved to an apartment, as she had not found a way to stay active and in her home. By giving up so many important things, she became more withdrawn and depressed. With the move, Dorothy became dependent on her son, who visited each week, for most of her support. She was not able to find a way to stay active in her church. She rarely shopped, and no longer attended any of her women's groups. These early and multiple losses happened even though Dorothy was very able to continue to participate. Dorothy's long-term outcomes were more negative than necessary because of her early withdrawal from activities.

The good news is that even with progressive memory loss you can take positive action to help maintain an active lifestyle. Even if you cannot remain totally independent, you can find ways to be active and engaged as you were in the past. Some of the basic guidelines that follow can help you find ways to stay active.

Focus on abilities—not losses

Too often, when people are diagnosed with progressive memory loss, they and their family members focus mainly on changes or losses. If you think mostly about what you have lost, you will find it hard to imagine how to stay active in the activities you have done in the past. You will limit your options, as you will be looking at the future in a very negative way. However, focusing on what you can still do rather than your losses allows you to find ways to stay active. You can use your retained abilities to your best advantage in finding ways to stay active and engaged. The positive story that you have just read is an example of focussing on abilities—not losses. Although Al was not as independent as he had been, by focusing on his abilities, he was able to be active.

Fit activities to match your abilities

Adapting an activity to match your abilities is a second way to help stay active. We described this method earlier in the chapter on maintaining your previous roles. Just by changing how you do something, you will be more likely to continue to do the activity. For example, if you can no longer plan long trips, you can still travel by going on short one- to two-day group outings. This way, you do not need to give up traveling—but just change the type of trip to match your ability to travel. Matching the activity to your level of ability will help you be successful in any activity.

Fit the environment to meet your needs

The third action that is helpful is to change your environment to help you function at your best. Some settings or environments may be hard for you to manage. For example, you may find busy shopping malls just too confusing for you to feel comfortable shopping. However, if you go to one department store that you are familiar with, you may still enjoy and feel comfortable shopping. Or, you may not be able to track the conversation if you are in a large group of people—but you still enjoy eating out and being with others. You can continue to be socially active just by limiting the number of people at any meeting or social event. Or, you may find you lose track of what someone is saying if the conversation is too long. It may be easier for you to function when you don't have to listen to someone talk for more than 5 or 10 minutes. You may find it helpful to arrange your environment to allow you to leave a conversation or talk if it is too long or hard for you to follow. You can change your home environment as well. To make it easier to do a task, for example, just keep the items you need close at hand. Or, make the appliances or tools easier to use. Try to use appliances that require only one or two steps to operate. You can also post a brief step-by-step list of instructions to help you use the technology (even cell phones) in your home. When you match your environment to your abilities, you can design activities that are safe and positive for you. You can also adapt your home or work environment to allow you to use technology and aids to help you function.

A variety of activities are available to people with memory loss to help you stay active and as independent as possible. Some activities are described below along with suggestions for how to make each activity work for you.

Work and volunteer activities

For people diagnosed with memory loss while still employed, staying active in work activities may be important to staying engaged. You and your employer may be able to work out ways for you to adapt your work to fit your abilities. This might include simplifying some of the tasks inherent in your work. You and your employer may also be able to find ways to modify the technology you use to make it easier for you. This might mean having step-by-step directions next to a computer or decreasing the number of steps needed to complete a work task. If you would feel more comfortable, you might ask your employer not to tell others about your diagnosis. In some work settings, however, your co-workers may be more understanding and supportive if they know why you are functioning somewhat differently in your work.

For people with memory loss who no longer work, volunteer activities may help you feel productive and assist in keeping you active. Volunteer activities can be found that match your ability and interests. Some communities have developed volunteer programs specifically for people with memory loss. These volunteer programs are developing across the USA and in other countries. Many of these programs match the volunteer with an appropriate activity and then pair the volunteer with someone else doing the same activity. Sometimes the second person is a student or older adult who also wishes to volunteer. Many of these volunteer positions are in museums, childcare centers, schools, hospitals, and social service agencies. These agencies often use volunteers to help carry out the work of the agency or for special projects. Volunteering in this type of agency helps to fulfill the goals and the work of the agency while providing you with a highly rewarding activity. If you are interested in volunteering, you might look for this type of opportunity in your own area. People who run volunteer programs for older adults with memory loss will help you match your abilities to the volunteer role. As long as you are physically and mentally able, volunteering may be a positive activity for you.

Driving

Changes in your ability to drive safely may be your biggest challenge to staying active and independent. However, being realistic about your driving ability may also prevent harm to both you and those around you. We know from research that even in the very early stages of memory loss a person with the loss is twice as likely to have an accident as someone without memory loss. This increase in risk of accidents is due to several changes in ability. One, your reaction time will be slowed. This slowed reaction time is caused by the increased processing time required with changes in your mental functioning. When driving, you will never know when you need to make a quick decision. Changes in your mental functioning make it harder for you to make that decision accurately and quickly enough to prevent an accident. The other change that occurs with memory loss is an altered ability to perceive the space around you accurately. For instance, you may have more difficulty estimating the distance between objects. So, you may not be able to perceive the distance between you and the car in front or behind you accurately. You may also not judge the space between cars while parking or pulling into a garage accurately. These changes increase your risk of hurting yourself and others while driving.

You can manage these changes in your ability to drive in a positive way. First, studies of driving suggest that you should have a driving evaluation at least every six months after your diagnosis of memory loss. This driving evaluation should be done with someone who is experienced in safe driving assessments, such as a licencing official or driving instructor. When it is difficult for you to be objective about your driving ability, this regular evaluation by a professional helps assure you that you are driving safely. Also, many healthcare providers for older adults administer safe driving examinations in their office. These non-driving tests are helpful, but are not as accurate as an actual driving evaluation. Both methods are ways to screen your ability to drive safely.

While changes in driving can be threatening to you, you may find positive ways to manage these changes in driving ability. Stopping driving does not necessarily mean that you will lose your independence. When you are no longer able to drive, you may want to let your family know that you want to be involved in decisions about how to replace your driving. Almost every community has support for transportation for people who are unable to drive. In an open and honest discussion with your family, you can let them know how you feel most comfortable getting around. You may decide you prefer to have family members or friends assist you in getting around. Or, you may prefer to use public transportation. The important part of this process is having a voice in how to stay active and replace your driving with other means of transportation.

You may also want to be part of a discussion about what to do with your automobile, if you own one. Many people with memory loss have described their anger if the family sells their car or removes it from their access without their knowledge. You may want to be part of that decision. Even if you cannot drive independently, you may want to keep your car for a short time just to see if there is some change in the future. One man with progressive memory loss I cared for, Ed, had been a truck driver most of his life. Even though he could no longer drive safely, Ed and his family decided to keep his car just in case there was a change in Ed's ability to drive. As Ed had been behind the wheel for many years, he would often go and sit in the car for several hours a day. Sitting behind the wheel of his car was comforting to Ed, and helped ease the transition to giving up driving. You may find other ways to help manage the loss of ability to drive. No matter how you stop driving, the important outcomes are for you to continue to be active and have a voice in how to maintain your activities.

Managing finances

Managing your finances can be one way you are able to stay independent. For years, you may have been the person to manage your finances on a day-to-day basis. Previously, you may have had no difficulty balancing your checkbook, paying bills, or keeping insurance coverage active. You may also have been the person to oversee your investments and financial health. One part of your mental ability that may be affected is your ability to manage your finances at the same level that you have in the past. Like driving, you may find it hard to be objective about your ability to continue to manage your finances. Being honest and open about your ability is important. If you are honest and pro-active, you will be more likely to prevent a mistake that can cause a financial loss for you or your family. However, the time may come when it becomes too difficult for you to manage your finances independently. Unfortunately, there are criminals who may recognize and take advantage of your difficulties with finances.

You may find it beneficial to work with your spouse or other family members to design some ways for you to stay involved in your financial affairs. For example, it may be difficult for you to balance your checkbook. You may want to let your spouse or other family members know that you want to be part of the bill-paying process. To stay involved in your financial management, you may work with your spouse or other family members to review the bills monthly and help make decisions about payments. If you cannot make decisions about your investments independently, you may still want to review your financial statements monthly and have a voice in how your money is invested.

You may also want to make it clear to your spouse or other family members that you would like to have some cash on hand. Often, family members become concerned that cash will be lost or spent for unneeded items because of the difficulty you are having with your memory. However, if it is important for you to have some cash, you will want to let others know that it is helpful to have cash available. You may need a minimal amount of cash for some last-minute items, such as bus or cab fare, personal items, a meal away from home, or supporting a fund drive if someone comes to the door—all the types of things you are used to paying for on a day-to-day basis. Keeping just a small amount of money on hand will prevent you from being concerned about losing large amounts of money or causing a financial hardship for others. Having a small amount of money available may also help you have the freedom to function as independently as possible.

Activities of daily living

Other common activities, called "activities of daily living," can be adapted to help you function as independently as possible. Activities like shopping, household tasks, or hobbies are common to most people with memory loss. These activities are generally carried out on a day-to-day basis. The types of daily activities each individual does will vary from person to person. For example, many women are involved with housekeeping tasks, while men may be more involved with home maintenance or yard work. Hobbies vary from person to person, depending on past interests and skills. The wide range of daily activities and hobbies prevents us from giving guidelines for each activity. However, some general guidelines will be given to help you find ways to adapt your daily activities to meet you abilities. The end of this chapter contains an example of how keeping a journal may help you find ways to stay active. You can use this journal to list the activities that you perform often. In one column, you can list the activity. In the second column, you can list ways to adapt the activity to allow you to continue with it. This simple guide will help you and your family members design ways for you to keep the activity in your routine.

When shopping becomes difficult for you, making changes in your shopping routine may help you continue to shop for yourself. For example, you may become more forgetful if you try to go to a number of different stores or shop for a number of different items at one time. Also, you may require some assistance with transportation. Requiring assistance to go to a store or shopping area does not mean you should give up shopping, however. You may want to go just to one place and shop for a few items at one time. You may also find it helpful to use reminders, such as a list, of all the items you need. You can refer to the list while shopping. If you need to shop in a large, crowded shopping mall or market, you might ask someone to go with you. Having a second person may help you feel more comfortable in crowded or confusing shopping areas or markets. You may also want to carry just enough money to pay for the items you want to purchase. By carrying only the cash you need or using only one credit card, you will lessen your chances of losing a credit card or overspending. If shopping for yourself is important and pleasant for you, try adapting how you shop to your abilities to help you stay active in shopping as long as possible.

Whether you are a male or female, you probably carry out some household tasks each day. The tasks often include outdoor work such as mowing, trimming bushes, woodworking, or caring for your home. Other daily indoor household tasks include cooking, cleaning, and laundry. All of these tasks can be broken down or simplified to allow you to perform them successfully. For example, when cooking, you may want to prepare meals that involve only one or two courses (such as meat and vegetable) rather than four or five courses (meat, vegetable, rice or potato, dessert). You may have no difficulty cooking one or two items, but may have trouble keeping up with three or four different items at the same time. You may want to use very simple recipes that have only a few ingredients. These simple recipes can be written in large print and posted at the meal preparation area. You will also want to make sure you allow enough time to prepare the meal. When you feel hurried or rushed, you will have more trouble thinking about what to do next. Allowing enough time to cook gives you the time to stop and think carefully about what step is next. Just making these simple changes in how you prepare a meal will make mealtime more enjoyable and safe.

With memory loss, you will find it difficult to complete more than one or two steps or actions at a time. Anytime you do household tasks, then, you will find it helpful to keep the task to one or two steps at the most at any one time. For example, if you are mowing your lawn, you will want to decide how to get the mower to where you want to start mowing: this is one step. When you get the mower to the right place, you think about what you need to do to start the mower: the second step. Once you start the mower, you might then decide on the pattern you want to take to mow: step three. If you break down any task into a step-by-step process, you are more likely to succeed in it. However, if you just think about everything you need to do to mow the lawn at once, the task may seem overwhelming to you.

Cleaning and laundry are tasks that are easy to break down into one or two steps. For example, cleaning can be broken down to one room at a time or one process at a time. You may first need to pick up items in the room and put them away: the first step. You may then decide to dust the room: a second step. You may then go back and vacuum the room after dusting: step three. Rather than thinking about everything you need to do to clean the entire house, try to do just one step in the cleaning process at a time. Limiting the cleaning to one area or room at a time is also helpful. Eventually, the entire house will be cleaned—one step at a time. Laundry can be done using the same process. You first might want to sort the laundry: step one. Next, you will put the cleaning agent into the washer: step two. Then, you can load the laundry: step three. You can then decide on the correct settings, thinking about only one setting at a time: step four. You may find it helpful to post this step-by-step list in the laundry area. That way, you can refer to the list to make sure you do not miss any steps in the laundry process. All of these very simple changes in your routine can help you stay active in the household tasks that you want to continue.

Hobbies are activities in which you may want to stay active and engaged. Some hobbies are more difficult to adapt with memory loss, such as woodworking, because of concerns about your safety. Other hobbies, such as gardening, can be more easily simplified and carried out safely. Again, breaking down the hobby into steps will help you do it with success. For example, you may no longer feel comfortable with the mechanics of plowing your garden space, so you may need to ask someone to plow your garden space for you. However, you can certainly do the planting and care for the garden. You can water and weed the garden, as well as gather any vegetables or flowers. Again, you might find it helpful to list each part of gardening into separate tasks. For planting, the tasks might include:

1. defining rows

2. digging the hole for plants or seeds

3. planting the seed or plant

4. covering the seed or root.

This type of list will help you stay "on task." Woodworking can be done using this same method. You may no longer feel comfortable using power tools safely, as safe usage requires paying close attention to a lot of different actions at the same time. But, you may feel comfortable using a hammer, sander, or hand tools. By using hand tools, you may continue to do woodworking projects.

One common hobby that many people enjoy is golf. Many people with memory loss become frustrated when they can no longer play 18 holes of golf. Not playing an entire 18 holes does not mean that you need to give up golfing entirely. You may continue golfing by playing short courses, such as par three courses or only nine holes. You can also go to driving ranges or putting greens to continue practicing and enjoying golf. The important outcome is that you are still golfing—a hobby you may have enjoyed much of your life. Most hobbies can continue to be a part of your life if you simplify the hobby to match your abilities. Also, remember to focus on what you are able to do rather than your losses when looking for ways to adapt the hobby.

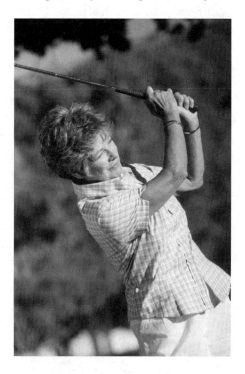

Benefits of adapting activities

You may be thinking that staying active in everything you have done in the past is not really that important to you. After all, you have new challenges each day that go along with progressive memory loss. You may think that you can give up golf or shopping and still enjoy your life. You may think you can give up your hobbies and still be the same person. These statements can certainly be true for you. However, if you stop doing a lot of the activities that were important to you in the past, you may lose what defines you as a unique person. You may also find yourself bored much of the time. With boredom, you may fall into a pattern called passive behavior. Research tells us that those people with memory loss who are more passive (less active) will have poorer long-term outcomes. Besides being bored, your mental and physical abilities may decline at a faster rate, as you are not using the mental and physical skills you have used before. While giving up one or two activities may not be negative, being less active in previous tasks and hobbies often results in negative outcomes.

Importantly, giving up activities is often not necessary. Many examples of adapting activities and hobbies to your abilities have been described in this chapter. Even if you are not able to do each activity or hobby as fully as you did in the past, continuing to do part of each activity will be positive. With a disease that affects your memory and mental ability, being creative and adapting the activities that mean the most to you are well worth the effort. Continuing to stay engaged in meaningful activities will have benefits for you years from now. So, the effort and energy you put into staying active now will be well worth the long-term benefits you will receive in years to come.

SAMPLE ACTIVITY JOURNAL

Activity/hobby	Steps to complete activity/ hobby	Ability
Example: 1. Pay bills	1. Gather all the bills in one place.	Organize
	2. Check date when payment is due.	
	3. Check balance in accounts.	Calculate
	4. Write or pay each bill one at a time.	Can write checks
	5. Place check and bill into envelope for mailing.	
	6. Have spouse or family member check payments before sending.	

YOUR ACTIVITY JOURNAL

Activity/hobby	Steps to complete activity/ hobby	Ability
1.	1.	
	2.	
	3.	
	4.	
	5.	
2.	1.	
	2.	
	3.	
	4.	
	5.	
3.	1.	
	2.	
	3.	
	4.	
	5.	
4.	1.	
	2.	
	3.	
	4.	
	5.	
5.	1.	
	2.	
	3.	
	4.	
	5.	

CHAPTER 7

Staying Physically Healthy: Managing Physical Illnesses, Medications, and Self-Care Needs

Many people with progressive memory loss have one or more other medical conditions. You need to continue to take care of your other medical conditions, in addition to your memory loss. This chapter will focus on taking care of yourself physically so that you can continue to feel good, do what you like to do, and remember and think as well as possible. This chapter is divided into a discussion of three health factors that may affect your memory and thinking:

1. physical illness

2. medications

3. self-care: nutrition and sleep.

Throughout the chapter, I will share several true stories about how these issues may affect people with progressive memory loss.

Physical illnesses

There are two types of physical illness: chronic and acute. *Chronic* illness refers to ongoing medical conditions, such as high blood pressure and diabetes. *Acute* illness refers to more sudden medical events, such as pneumonia or urinary tract infection. Both chronic and acute illness can worsen thinking and memory in people with progressive memory loss.

Chronic illness

You may have one of more of the following common medical conditions: arthritis, high blood pressure, diabetes, osteoporosis, emphysema, urinary problems, or a variety of heart problems. You may even have other conditions that are not on this list. Chronic medical conditions require lifelong monitoring and treatment to control symptoms and prevent complications. Good medical care for chronic medical conditions is particularly important for people with progressive memory loss because physical problems can worsen mental functioning.

Many chronic medical conditions are associated with worsening mental functioning. For example, high blood pressure, high cholesterol, high blood sugar, thyroid problems, and poor kidney function may all worsen thinking and memory. Good treatment of these medical conditions may improve memory and thinking, in addition to extending your life.

Acute illness

When people with progressive memory loss become acutely ill, the illness itself can make their memory problems much worse. This is called "delirium" [di-*leer*-ee-uhm] or "acute confusion." Any person, of any age, can experience delirium if he or she becomes ill enough. However, delirium during physical illness occurs more often among older adults who already have memory loss. This means that it is even more important for you to keep as physically healthy as possible now that you are having memory problems.

Experiencing delirium or acute confusion could mean that you are physically ill, even if the only symptom you have is increased confusion. For example, you could have a urinary tract (bladder or kidney) infection and not feel ill in any way. You may only feel much more confused. If you or your family or friends notice that your memory and thinking is suddenly much worse, this change could be delirium. Progressive memory loss is usually a very slow process. A sudden change in your thinking and memory is more likely to be caused by a physical illness. Do not assume that your memory and thinking are suddenly worse just because of your diagnosis of progressive memory loss. You should always seek medical care for sudden changes in your thinking and memory.

Below is a list of common causes of delirium or acute confusion.

1. Urinary tract infection (bladder or kidney infection).

2. Respiratory infection (colds, bronchitis, pneumonia).

3. Dehydration (too little water in the body).

4. Medications (discussed in more detail later in this chapter).

5. Blood sugar being too high or too low.

6. Severe constipation.

If you are physically ill and develop delirium, your behavior could become either very agitated or very sluggish. Other people, including some healthcare providers, could make a mistake and think your behavior is deliberately " difficult". Healthcare providers and others can also see your behavior as just a natural result of your memory loss. The appropriate treatment for delirium is for your healthcare provider to find and treat the cause of your increased confusion. After the cause has been treated, then the delirium will clear. For example, if you have delirium or acute confusion because of an infection, treating the infection with antibiotics will clear the delirium. Your thinking and memory will improve to the level it was before you developed the infection. It may take a few days or a few weeks for delirium to completely clear after the cause has been treated.

Unfortunately for some persons with delirium, their agitation may *not* be understood as being caused by physical illness. A healthcare provider might give sedating (calming) medications, instead of finding and correcting the real problem. Sometimes during delirium, sedating medications may be needed for your safety and comfort. However, delirium or acute confusion should never be treated *only* with sedatives. It is very important that you, with help from your family and/or your friends, seek medical attention if you have sudden, worsening confusion.

The next two stories are real and happened to people with memory loss. The first story is of a woman, Jane, who developed delirium. In Jane's case, her delirium was accurately diagnosed and treated. In the second story, Jim's story, the delirium was not diagnosed until it was necessary for Jim to be admitted to the hospital. In Jim's case, the result of not diagnosing delirium caused Jim much more physical pain and loss of function than if the delirium had been diagnosed sooner.

Jane's story

Jane had mild or early progressive memory loss. She was still able to live alone with help from her family and friends. Jane's daughter visited her every evening after work. One evening, Jane was very confused and did not even recognize her daughter. Fortunately, Jane's daughter realized that something was very wrong and she took her mother to the hospital. Jane had a urinary tract infection that was successfully treated with antibiotics. Jane's daughter thought it was strange that her mother never complained about any urinary problems even though she had an infection. Jane's daughter did not understand that older adults with memory loss may forget to tell others of their symptoms. People with memory loss are also often not listened to when they do complain, so they will stop telling others of their symptoms after a while. Older adults also may not have a fever or high temperature with an infection, as younger people do. All of these reasons may have made it harder for Jane's daughter to know about Jane's infection. Many people with progressive memory loss may have increased confusion or delirium as the main symptom of a physical illness. It took a few weeks for Jane to return to her previous level of functioning and "feel as good as new."

Jim's story

Jim was a 75-year-old retired factory worker who lived in an assisted living facility. Jim was able to care for himself entirely. He was generally very happy and took part in a number of different activities at the facility. One Monday, Jim became distressed and had more difficulty dressing and eating than he had a few days earlier. Jim's healthcare provider mistook his change in function as increased memory loss and put Jim on a sedating medication. With each passing day, Jim became worse and his confusion increased. As the healthcare provider still did not recognize Jim's change in behavior as acute confusion or delirium, the dose of Jim's sedating medications was increased. Finally, at the end of the week, a very caring nursing assistant decided to check Jim for a urinary tract infection. The nursing assistant knew that Jim's memory problems would not have increased so fast and that his symptoms were caused by a medical problem. By the time the nursing assistant found Jim's urinary tract infection, he was so sick he needed to be admitted to the local hospital for treatment. If Jim's healthcare provider or family had recognized that his change in mental ability was acute confusion or delirium, he could have received the proper diagnosis and treatment much sooner. Jim's life was at risk because of the delay in getting a proper diagnosis and treatment for the cause of his delirium.

Medications

Good medication management is particularly important for you, because of your progressive memory loss. Good medical care for chronic and acute illnesses can help to maintain your memory and thinking. Good medical care for physical illnesses, however, often requires medications. If you have many medical conditions, you may be taking many medications. Medications themselves can sometimes be a cause of increased confusion or delirium. So what is the right amount and type of medication for you? Only your healthcare provider can weigh the risks and benefits of particular medications for you. However, I will give you some general information about medications that everyone with progressive memory loss needs to know.

The cholinergic theory

The cholinergic (koh-luh-*nur*-jik) theory explains what helps memory and thinking in the brain, and what happens to people with progressive memory loss. There is a chemical in the brain called acetylcholine (uh-seet-l-*koh*-leen). Acetylcholine helps keep the brain cells communicating with each other, and thus promotes better thinking and memory. People with progressive memory loss have changes in the amount and functioning of acetylcholine in the brain. So medications that increase acetylcholine in the brain are generally good for people with progressive memory loss.

Another chemical in the brain that naturally breaks down acetylcholine is called cholinesterase (koh-luh-*nes*-tuh-reys). One category of medications used to treat people with memory loss is called cholinesterase inhibitors. Cholinesterase inhibitors interfere with or block cholinesterase. Because there is less cholinesterase to break down acetylcholine, there is more acetylcholine around the brain cells. Making acetylcholine more available in the brain is how cholinesterase inhibitors help with thinking and memory.

There are many medications that have anticholinergic (an-ti-koh-luh-*nur*-jik) side effects. These medications block the action of acetylcholine in the brain and can then interfere with thinking and memory even in people without memory problems. In individuals who already have memory loss, the effects of anticholinergic medications can be even more negative to thinking and memory. In general, people with progressive memory loss should avoid medications with anticholinergic side effects. Anticholinergic medications will be discussed in more detail later in this chapter.

Medications to treat progressive memory loss

Although the medications used to treat memory loss will be briefly described here, you should consult your healthcare provider about the possible risks and benefits of the medications for you. There are currently two basic types of medications available to treat progressive memory loss.

1. Cholinesterase inhibitors:

    (a) tacrine (brand name: Cognex)—no longer used

    (b) donepezil (brand name: Aricept)

    (c) galantamine (brand name: Razadyne, formerly called Reminyl)

    (d) rivastigmine (brand name: Exelon)

2. NMDA-receptor antagonist:

(a) memantine (brand name: Namenda)

The cholinesterase inhibitors were the first type of medication available to treat progressive memory loss. Cognex was the first drug in this class, but this drug is no longer routinely used because it had many side effects. The other three drugs, Aricept, Exelon, and Razadyne, are widely used. Some healthcare providers may have a preference for one of these medications instead of the others. However, all three medications work about the same, with some very minor differences. All of these medications work by blocking the chemical that breaks down acetylcholine and thus can increase the amount of acetylcholine in the brain. The increased levels of acetylcholine in the brain help to slow down the memory and thinking changes that occur with progressive memory loss. Cholinesterase inhibitors are approved for the treatment of persons with mild to moderate dementia or progressive memory loss. These medications tend to work best when started very soon after memory loss begins. The medications are generally continued until the person can no longer benefit. The medications do not cure memory loss, but slow down the decline in memory loss and function.

The second category of medications for treating progressive memory loss, the NMDA-receptor antagonist, has only one drug at this time: memantine (brand name: Namenda). Namenda works in an entirely different way than the cholinesterase inhibitors. There is another chemical messenger in the brain called glutamate. Glutamate is also important for memory and thinking. However, if glutamate levels are too high, brain cells may be damaged and unable to function well. Namenda works by helping to protect the brain cells from high levels of glutamate. Because Namenda and the cholinesterase inhibitors work differently, the two types of medications can be combined safely. Taking both medications together provides more benefit than taking either medication separately. Namenda is approved for the treatment of people with moderate to severe dementia or progressive memory loss. Namenda does not cure memory loss, but helps to slow down the decline in memory and function.

Here are some common questions that people with progressive memory loss often have about the medications.

1. *When should medications for progressive memory loss be started?* Most healthcare providers recommend starting cholinesterase inhibitors as soon as the diagnosis is confirmed. Namenda is often added to the cholinesterase inhibitor at a later time. Although the medications work better together than alone, starting both medications at the same time is not usually recommended.

2. *What are the side effects of the medications for progressive memory loss?* For the cholinesterase inhibitors, the most common side effects are stomach upset, nausea, diarrhea, and poor appetite. For memantine, the most common side effects are dizziness, headache, and constipation. Usually, the medications are started at very low doses and gradually increased. This helps lessen the side effects. Occasionally, people with progressive memory loss experience a feeling of "awakening" or slight agitation when first taking the medications. If this happens, the dose of the medication can be lowered temporarily. In general, medications for progressive memory loss are very well tolerated compared to many other medications.

3. *How do we know that medications for progressive memory loss are working?* It usually takes several months of continuous treatment with the medications to see any benefits. You may only notice that you are not getting any worse over a period of time. Without taking the medication, we know that the symptoms get worse over time. If your memory and function stay about the same over several months, then the medications are probably working for you.

4. *When should medications for progressive memory loss be stopped?* In general, once the medications have been started, they should not be stopped until there is no longer a benefit. Healthcare providers, families, and insurers may all differ in their opinions about how long to continue the medications. It is probably best to discuss these differences honestly and openly. The benefit of the medications is that thinking and functioning will be better for a longer period of time. If you are taking the medications, you are expected to be able to care for yourself longer than if you were not taking the medications.

5. *Are the medications for progressive memory loss worth the cost?* Probably, yes. When the costs of providing care for people with progressive memory loss are considered, the costs of the medications to help you continue to care for yourself are much less.

6. *Should the medications for progressive memory loss be stopped for illness or during hospitalization?* Generally, no. Suddenly stopping medications for memory loss can worsen function. Restarting the medications after a long delay may not return you to the same level of function. If you are unable to take the medications for a few days because of severe illness, it is important to restart them as soon as possible.

Obviously, if your illness was caused by the medications, then they should be stopped. However, it is rare for these medications to cause severe side effects that require stopping the medication.

If you want to find out more about medications for progressive memory loss, ask your healthcare provider and/or pharmacist. A great deal of research is currently being done to find new and even better medications to treat progressive memory loss. An example of what medication can achieve follows below.

John's story

John was diagnosed with early or mild progressive memory loss after taking several memory tests. His healthcare provider prescribed a cholinesterase inhibitor, donepezil (brand name: Aricept). John began taking the medication at a low dose. He complained of some mild nausea for a few weeks but then the nausea went away. After about six weeks he began taking a higher dose of the medication. John had been hoping to feel a lot different and mentally sharper on the medication but he really didn't notice much difference. John's wife said she thought he might be doing a little better. After taking the medication for six months, John repeated the same memory tests. The tests showed that his memory and thinking were about the same as when he had started the medication. John was very disappointed that the medication had not helped him. Medications for progressive memory loss slow the expected changes. John's medication is helping him because without the medication, he would be expected to be worse after six months. Instead, John has been able to maintain his memory and function over the six-month period while taking the medication.

As John's memory loss progressed, his healthcare provider decided to add memantine (Namenda). Again the medication was started at a low dose and gradually increased. John continued to take donepezil (brand name: Aricept) also. John's wife thought that he might be a little too agitated on the new medication so his dose was temporarily decreased and then increased again as he adjusted to the medication. John has been on both medications now for two years. His memory and thinking have gradually worsened but not as much as if he had not been taking the medications. The medications are helping to keep John at home with his wife.

Other medications

You may be taking one or more medications for your medical conditions, in addition to taking medication for your memory. Taking many different medications increases your risk of having medication side effects. People with progressive memory loss are more likely to have central nervous system (brain) side effects such as sleepiness, confusion, and agitation from medications.

For people with progressive memory loss, one of the worst categories of medications is what we call "anticholinergic" [anti-co-lin-er-jic] medications. Many common medications, both prescribed and over-the-counter (OTC), are classified as anticholinergic. There is a good reason why these drugs are generally considered the worst for people with memory loss. A chemical in the brain called acetylcholine [ass-a-tyl-ko-leen] helps with memory and thinking. When you take a medication with anticholinergic side effects, acetylcholine is blocked and you can become more confused. Also, many other possible negative side effects of anticholinergic medications exist, including drowsiness, constipation, dry eyes, dry mouth, difficulty urinating (passing urine), difficulty perspiring even when very overheated, and changing blood pressure, which may cause falls. For people with progressive memory loss who are taking cholinesterase inhibitors (like Aricept), it makes no sense at all to be taking anticholinergic medications. The two types of medications would be working at cross-purposes, each canceling out the effects of the other. It is important to avoid anticholinergic medications if at all possible. You should ask your primary healthcare provider and/or pharmacist to regularly review a list of the medications you are taking. You might want to write something like this statement at the top of your medication list: "I have progressive memory loss. Please help me to avoid taking medications with anticholinergic side effects, if at all possible. I want to continue to think and remember as well as possible for as long as possible."

Table 7.1 on the next page lists common anticholinergic medications. This list is not complete. Many other medications have anticholinergic side effects.

The benzodiazepines or anti-anxiety medications are another group of medications that often causes problems for people with progressive memory loss. Some examples of anti-anxiety medications are: lorazepam (brand name: Ativan), alprazolam (brand name: Xanax), temazepam (brand name: Restoril). These anti-anxiety medications, sometimes used for sleep problems, can cause increased confusion and falls in people with progressive memory loss. If you feel very anxious or nervous, you should be carefully evaluated by a specialist (psychiatrist or psychologist) before asking for or taking anti-anxiety medications. Most persons with progressive memory loss will function better if they do *not* take anti-anxiety medications. Sometimes other medications, like antidepressants, can help treat anxiety with fewer side effects. Medications need careful consideration, as Mary's story shows.

Table 7.1 Common anticholinergic medications

Generic name	Possible trade names	Used for
Amitriptyline	Elavil	Depression/sleep problems/pain
Cimetidine	Tagamet	Indigestion
Cyclobenzaprine	Flexeril	Muscle spasms
Diphenhydramine	Benadryl	Allergies
	Tylenol PM*	Sleep problems
Dicyclomine	Bentyl	Intestinal spasms/diarrhea
Meclizine	Antivert, Bonine	Dizziness
Oxybutynin	Ditropan	Bladder spasms

*Tylenol PM is a combination of acetaminophen (Tylenol) and diphenhydramine.
Acetaminophen is safe and effective for people with progressive memory loss so long as the recommended dosage is taken. Diphenhydramine, however, is very anticholinergic and should not be taken by people with progressive memory loss. Diphenhydramine is the active ingredient in many over the counter (OTC) sleeping medications.

Mary's story

Mary had progressive memory loss, and was living with her daughter. She had some history of dizziness and had been taking meclizine (Antivert) for several years even though it did not seem to help her dizziness much. She was also taking several medications for high blood pressure, though she had not had her blood pressure checked for several months. One evening, her daughter took Mary to the emergency room of the local hospital because she was complaining of severe leg cramps. Although no cause for her leg cramps could be determined, Mary was given a prescription for amitriptyline (Elavil), a medication that is sometimes used for leg pain. Taking the amitriptyline (Elavil) made her more confused and drowsy, even during the day. She was not eating and drinking as much as usual. One day, she decided to go with some friends to a local ice cream parlor. The summer weather was very hot. While at the ice cream parlor, she suddenly collapsed, broke her arm and shoulder, and suffered a concussion.

What happened to Mary? At first glance, this might just seem like one of those unavoidable accidents that happen to older people. However, this accident most likely could have been prevented. Here's what I think happened to Mary and how it could have been prevented. Mary had been taking meclizine (Antivert) for a long time, even though it wasn't helping her much. Antivert is a highly anticholinergic drug that can cause dizziness, sleepiness, confusion, and sudden drops in blood pressure. Mary may have been just barely tolerating this drug for a long time. Mary was also taking medications to treat her high blood pressure but she wasn't being carefully monitored. Amitriptyline (Elavil) was added recently. This medication may also cause dizziness, weakness, sudden drops in blood pressure, and falls. Anticholinergic medications, like Elavil and Antivert, also decrease the ability to perspire or sweat. All of these factors came together on a hot day and Mary fell.

What could have been done differently? Mary should not have been taking anticholinergic medications. Unfortunately, not all healthcare providers know about this subject. Mary and her daughter could have asked more questions about her medications. The pharmacist is a very good resource for answering questions about medications. Mary was taking her blood pressure medications but was not having her blood pressure checked regularly and it may have been too low, causing her to fall. Mary admitted to feeling more sleepy and confused. She may not have been drinking enough fluids. Finally, because of increased sleepiness and confusion from the medications, Mary may have been taking some of her medications incorrectly. For Mary, taking too many of the wrong medications led to a lot of pain and expense that could have been prevented. Medication side effects can cause increased confusion (delirium) and falls, particularly in people with progressive memory loss. People with progressive memory loss must be very careful about taking medications. Don't be afraid to ask questions about your medications. Your healthcare provider and/or pharmacist can answer your questions about medications.

Self-care needs: nutrition and supplements

In general, people with progressive memory loss should eat the same balanced diet that would be recommended for any adult of about the same age. Keeping your weight around the ideal weight for your height will help you maintain your strength and endurance. You should weigh yourself at home on a regular basis, about once a month, keep track of your weight, and inform your healthcare provider of any changes in your weight. If you have recently been gaining or losing weight or have certain heart problems, you may need to weigh yourself more often than once a month.

At times, people with progressive memory loss may suffer from appetite problems. Poor appetite is a side effect of many medications, including some of the medications taken for memory loss (like cholinesterase inhibitors). Once cholinesterase inhibitors have been taken for several weeks, the appetite problems usually get better. Poor appetite may also be caused by depression. If you or your family members notice that your appetite is poor or that you are losing weight without dieting, you need to have a thorough evaluation by your healthcare provider. Poor appetite is often treated first by stopping the medications that cause the problem. If necessary, medications that help to increase appetite may be added. If weight loss continues, your healthcare provider may add a nutritious drink or snack to your daily diet. It is important to keep your weight as normal as possible. Continuous weight loss weakens the immune system and makes you more vulnerable to acute illnesses. On the other hand, if you weigh too much, you will not be able to be as physically active as you need to be. Before trying to diet to lose weight, be sure to talk to your healthcare provider.

Low levels of vitamin B12 or folate may worsen memory and thinking problems. Your primary healthcare provider can check to see if your vitamin B12 or folate level is too low with a simple blood test. If your levels are low, you can take vitamin B12 or folate supplements, or both. Antioxidants are vitamins that tend to protect cells, including brain cells, from a sort of natural damage (oxidative damage) that occurs over time as we age. Vitamin C, vitamin E, and beta carotene are all examples of antioxidants. One of the best ways to get enough antioxidants in your diet is to eat a variety of fresh fruits and vegetables every day. If you are thinking about taking anything more than a multivitamin once a day, you should consult your healthcare provider. Large doses of some vitamins may be more harmful than helpful.

Gingko biloba is taken by some people with progressive memory loss as a way to improve memory. The evidence for the effectiveness of gingko biloba for memory loss is not clear. However, taking gingko biloba in combination with other drugs, especially anticoagulants or blood thinners, can be dangerous. Again, the safest thing to do is to ask your healthcare provider before taking gingko biloba or any other herbal substance. Do not take any vitamin or herbal supplements without checking with your healthcare provider first.

One of the most important nutritional substances is plain water. Many people, with or without memory loss, do not drink enough fluids. For individuals with progressive memory loss, becoming dehydrated (not having enough water in the body) is likely to increase confusion and cause delirium. Poor fluid intake may also worsen bowel and bladder function. Ask your healthcare provider about how much fluid you need to be drinking every day. A general guideline is to drink about one ounce of fluid per day for every two pounds body weight. For example, if you weigh 110 pounds, you would need about 55 ounces of fluid daily. If you are overweight, use your ideal body weight to calculate your fluid needs. Water is one of the best fluids to drink. Beverages with caffeine are not as beneficial as caffeine acts like a mild diuretic or "water pill." If you have specific health conditions, you may need to limit your fluid intake. Do not limit your fluid intake unless you have been told to do so by your healthcare provider. Bob's story shows the importance of finding the right medication.

Bob's story

Bob had early progressive memory loss. He had been taking a cholinesterase inhibitor, galantamine (brand name: Razadyne), for about one year without any major problems. Bob started feeling less hungry and he noticed that he was losing weight, even though he was not dieting. Bob made an appointment to see his healthcare provider. After reviewing his medication list, Bob's healthcare provider stopped several medications that could be decreasing his appetite. Although cholinesterase inhibitors can sometimes cause poor appetite and weight loss when first started, it is not likely that Bob would develop this side effect after taking the medication for a year. His healthcare provider continued the Razadyne because it was helping Bob's memory and function. Bob's appetite returned and he maintained his weight for the next year. After about a year, Bob's appetite worsened again and he began to have difficulty sleeping and to lose interest in his regular activities. Again, he made an appointment to see his healthcare provider, who thought that Bob might be depressed. Depression is common in people with progressive memory loss. Bob saw a psychiatrist who started an antidepressant medication for him. The antidepressant helped his mood, appetite, and sleep. Bob continues to live at home and is enjoying life even more now that his depression has been successfully treated. He has resumed playing golf several days a week.

Self-care needs: sleep

Many people with progressive memory loss complain about poor sleep. Some of the common complaints are:

1. difficulty getting to sleep

2. awakening frequently during the night

3.   awakening too early in the morning

4.   feeling overly tired during the day.

It is important to understand that sleep patterns change naturally with aging, even in people who do not have memory loss. Increased sleep problems with aging are one of those unfair changes that happen in life: 50-, 60-, or 70-year-old people *cannot* expect to sleep better than they did when they were 20 or 30 years old. A natural response to this situation is to take a sleep medication to help you sleep better and longer. However, most sleep medications should *not* be taken by people with progressive memory loss.

Most sleep medications available without a prescription generally contain diphenhydramine (brand name: Benadryl). This medication can cause increased confusion and other bad side effects in people with progressive memory loss. Many sleep medications that are available with a prescription are called benzodiazepines. These are medications like temazepam (brand name: Restoril). Benzodiazepines can increase confusion and falls in people with progressive memory loss. Unfortunately, most sleep medications have too many bad side effects to be taken safely by people with progressive memory loss. Also, even when sleep medications help with sleep for a few nights, over time, the quality of sleep generally worsens when using the sleep medications. The opposite of what you might expect actually happens: the longer that you take a sleep medication, the less likely you are to sleep well! If you need to use a sleep medication once in a while, then it is likely to work for you. However, taking sleep medications every night generally results in chronic poor sleep. Sleep medications may also cause hangover effects. The day after taking a sleep medication, you may feel drowsy and confused. There are some newer sleep medications that have fewer bad side effects. Before trying any sleep medications, though, it would be better to try some non-medication ways to improve your sleep. The following is a list of things you can try if you are having trouble sleeping.

1.   Go to bed a little later in the evening. You will sleep longer into the night. If you only need about eight hours of sleep and you go to bed at eight o'clock in the evening, then your body will be done sleeping by about four o'clock in the morning. This is not insomnia. The solution to this problem is to gradually stay up a little later each night until you have reached a bedtime and awakening time that works for you.

2. Try to maintain a regular sleep schedule. Go to bed and get up about the same time every day. Try to keep your sleep schedule the same even on weekends and holidays.

3. Exercise in the morning or early afternoon. Staying active promotes better sleep. However, if you exercise too late in the day, you may have more trouble getting to sleep at night.

4. Develop a bedtime routine: a light snack, a warm bath, soothing music. Try whatever relaxes you. If you eat something before bedtime, keep it light. Heavy meals before bed can disrupt sleep. Tryptophan (found in milk and turkey) is a natural chemical that can help you sleep. Your mother and grandmother were right: warm milk really can help you sleep better!

5. Keep your bed for sleep and romantic activities only. Do not do other activities in bed. If you do activities in bed, you are training your body to be active in bed, rather than restful in bed. Do not watch television in bed. Watch television somewhere else until you are tired and then go to bed.

6. Make your bed and bedroom a good place to sleep. For most people, this will be a quiet, dark, cooler room. Invest in a new mattress if needed. Pamper yourself a little with comfortable sheets, blankets, and pillows.

7. Do not use alcohol as a sleep medication. Alcoholic beverages may make you sleepy and help you go to sleep, however, alcohol causes sleep problems during the night. If you drink an alcoholic beverage just before sleep, you are likely to awaken a few hours later, need to urinate, and be unable to return to sleep. If your healthcare provider approves and you wish to have an alcoholic drink in the evening, it is better to have the drink earlier, for example, at six o'clock in the evening. This should not interfere with your sleep.

8. Avoid stimulants like nicotine and caffeine. If you want to drink tea, coffee, or soft drinks with caffeine, do so earlier in the day, before noon, if possible. If you smoke, try to stop. Nicotine in tobacco disrupts sleep and makes your overall health poorer. If you cannot quit smoking completely, avoid smoking in the evening before bedtime.

9. If you have been in bed for more than about 20 minutes and cannot fall asleep, get out of bed. Do not go back to bed until you

are tired. If you do not fall asleep until late at night, you should still try to get out of bed at the same time in the morning. You will be more tired and ready to fall asleep the next night.

10. If you take a nap in the afternoon, keep it short, no longer than about 30–60 minutes. Longer naps are likely to interfere with your nighttime sleep. Also, if you must take an afternoon nap, take the nap before three o'clock or so in the afternoon. Later afternoon naps are more likely to cause you to have trouble sleeping at night.

11. Ask your healthcare provider to review your medication list for medications that might be worsening your sleep. If you have been taking a sleep medication regularly for a long time, you may have to gradually decrease and stop the sleep medication in order to sleep better. Do *not* suddenly stop taking sleep medications on your own. In some cases, this can be dangerous. Talk to your healthcare provider about stopping sleep medications.

12. If you have tried the above ideas and are still have trouble sleeping, you may need to have a more thorough sleep evaluation. This evaluation is usually conducted by a specialist in sleep problems. You will be monitored for a night while you sleep to make sure that you don't have a physical problem, such as difficulty breathing, interfering with your sleep.

13. If you do need a sleep medication, some of the newer sleep medications or an antidepressant medication that promotes sleep may be safer for you. Your healthcare provider will need to consider the risks and benefits of these medications for you.

In Elizabeth's story on the next page, non-medication solutions proved more positive for her than medication. Many sleep medications can worsen memory and thinking in people with progressive memory loss.

What's the point?

Some people with progressive memory loss have asked me: "What's the point of taking care of myself physically if my mind is deteriorating?" You may have asked yourself or others a similar question. This sensitive topic is worth discussing honestly. Some people with memory loss may feel that it is better to neglect their physical health because they would rather die before they reach the later stages of progressive memory loss. Unfortunately, some healthcare providers and health policy makers may share this view. Healthcare providers may

Elizabeth's story

Elizabeth has progressive memory loss. She has always considered herself a somewhat nervous person. For several years, Elizabeth has taken lorazepam (brand name: Ativan) for her "nerves" and temazepam (brand name: Restoril) for her sleep problems. The medications don't seem to be helping her much anymore. Elizabeth made an appointment with her healthcare provider. She requested a higher dose of Restoril to help her sleep better. Elizabeth was upset when her healthcare provider explained that she would feel better and sleep better if she stopped taking benzodiazepine medications like Ativan and Restoril. Her healthcare provider explained that she would need to gradually decrease these medications. Stopping these medications too quickly can be dangerous. While gradually decreasing her sleep medications, Elizabeth tried several of the same non-medication ideas we have already discussed. At first, Elizabeth's sleep was worse. However, after a few weeks her sleep improved, and she felt more rested during the day. She was no longer taking any sleep medications. An additional benefit for Elizabeth was that her mind felt clearer than when she had been taking the sleep medications.

routinely deny certain types of necessary medical care to individuals just because they have progressive memory loss. Based on experience in caring for people with memory loss, I do not agree that not treating physical health problems is an appropriate choice.

Many of my older clients, even those without progressive memory loss, express the desire to be completely healthy until the time of death. They might wish to go to sleep and just not wake up again the next day. I think many of us wish for that sort of life and death. The reality, however, is that very few people will die suddenly due to poor health. Instead, neglecting your health is much more likely to cause uncomfortable symptoms, a loss of functioning, more visits to the physician, and more time in the hospital. If you neglect healthcare for a condition such as diabetes or high blood pressure, you will not necessarily pass away more quickly. You will, however, have many more complications that worsen your physical and mental functioning. Not caring for your health can reduce your quality of life when you might otherwise live in comfort.

In general, the fact that you have progressive memory loss should not make you any less likely to receive most medical treatments. At times, you may be treated in a slightly different manner for a particular medical condition because of your progressive memory loss. The healthcare provider, after talking with you and your family members, must weigh the potential risks and benefits of treatments for you. For example, some older adults have urinary leakage problems. Medications are available that can help this condition, but some of the medications could make your memory loss and confusion worse. In this case, your healthcare provider might decide that the risk of the medication is greater than the benefit of the medication for you.

You and your family or friends should visit your healthcare provider on a regular basis to discuss your health and the plan of care. By treating all of your medical conditions appropriately, you will be able to enjoy your life more in the here and now. At the end of this chapter is a self-care guide. You can use this guide to help you plan for your own care. You can also use the guide to remind you of steps you can take to protect your health. Some people with progressive memory loss spend a lot of time and energy thinking about what might happen to them in the future. Although it is important for all individuals, of any age, to plan ahead in life, enjoying life now is just as important. We are all going to die someday, of something. As my father used to say, "None of us are getting out of here alive!" In that sense, people with progressive memory loss are not facing a future any different from everyone else. Your future will be brighter and more comfortable if you receive proper care for your medical illnesses.

SELF-CARE GUIDE (1)

- Make sure you have one primary healthcare provider—someone who knows everything about your health. If you need to see specialists, make sure the specialists and your primary healthcare provider talk to you and each other about your care. Having too many healthcare providers can be a problem, especially if they are not communicating well.

- See your healthcare provider on a regular basis to prevent and treat illnesses.

- Most, if not all, of your illnesses should be treated the same as if you did not have progressive memory loss. If someone tries to deny you healthcare based on your memory loss, ask them to explain why you are being treated differently.

- At home, keep a running list of problems and questions that you have for your healthcare provider. Take that list of questions to all of your appointments. Write down the answers to your questions during your appointment. You might want to keep this as a type of diary with dated entries.

- Enlist a family member or close friend to be your healthcare advocate. Ask this person to go to healthcare provider appointments with you. Don't feel embarrassed about including a healthcare advocate in your care. Everyone, even people without memory problems, needs help to get through the healthcare system with success.

- Keep an updated list of all of your medications with you at all times. Make sure that a family member or friend also has the medication list.

- Take your medication list to every appointment with your healthcare provider. Discuss the medication list with your healthcare provider. If medication changes are made, make sure the change is noted on your list.

- Do not take any over-the-counter (OTC) medications, vitamins, or herbal supplements without the consent of your primary healthcare provider.

SELF-CARE GUIDE (2)

- Understand that adding another medication is not always the best solution to a problem. Sometimes stopping a medication you are already taking may be better for you. Some of your symptoms (e.g. increased confusion, dizziness, falls) may actually be caused by a medication you are taking.

- Work with your healthcare provider to solve some of your health problems with something other than more medications. For example, a warm bath and gentle stretching exercises may help joint pain. A glass of warm milk at bedtime may help you sleep.

- Take all of your medications as prescribed by your healthcare provider.

- Take care of your general health: eat well, balance your rest and activity, and drink plenty of fluids.

- If you notice that your memory or thinking is suddenly worse, see your healthcare provider immediately. Remember, changes in memory or thinking occur very slowly in progressive memory loss. *Rapid changes* in memory, thinking, or your behavior are probably caused by an illness that needs to be treated *right away*.

- Plan for the future but don't dwell on your future. Instead, enjoy living each day to the fullest.

CHAPTER 8

Staying Mentally Healthy: Managing Memory Loss and Impaired Thinking

Illnesses that cause memory loss and impaired thinking are often progressive in nature. However, as we discussed in the previous chapter on maintaining physical health, treatments, other than medications, are available to help boost your mental health and wellbeing. The old saying "use it or lose it" is just as true for your memory or brain "muscle" as it is for other muscles in your body. Just as it is important is to keep exercising muscles in our body, exercising your brain can help with mental fitness. In this chapter, treatments and activities designed to exercise your brain will be described. These treatments may help you maintain your memory and mental abilities.

When you think about treatments for progressive memory loss, the most common treatment is medications. Non-medication treatments and activities are often not suggested or prescribed by your healthcare provider, although studies have shown many other treatments may be helpful. Combining medications with non-medication treatments increases the strength or power of the total treatment. Although results of treatment will vary from person to person, a more powerful treatment should result in greater benefits for your mental functioning. Even in a disease that causes progressive memory loss, focussing on wellness and exercising your body and brain may help slow the loss.

Benefits of non-medication treatments
Self-care
In addition to helping maintain mental functioning, non-medication treatments can have other benefits for you. Participating in non-medication treatments gives you the chance to do something for yourself. When taking medications, you are also doing something for yourself. But, the medications are prescribed. You have little choice over the kinds of medications you take and how they are taken. With non-medication treatments, you can decide what types of treatments and activities are right for you. You can find activities that meet your own individual needs. So, with non-medication treatments, you have

some choice in the treatment—giving you more control over your total care. By choosing the treatments that fit your interests and strengths, you are more likely to have positive results for your mental functioning.

Normal living

Many types of non-medication treatments and activities are part of normal living. Often people with memory loss have told me that they want very much for their life to go back to normal. Normal, before your diagnosis, may have been walking three times a week, taking part in art classes, being part of social clubs and groups, or dancing weekly with your spouse at a dance club. You do not need to stop these activities because of your diagnosis of progressive memory loss. Some of these activities can actually promote your mental health and functioning. If you have never engaged in these activities before, now may be the time to start. Starting these non-medication activities and treatments may help you feel more normal, while improving your mental functioning.

Social support

Non-medication treatments often include social activities. In non-medication treatments such as exercise or dance groups you are increasing your social contacts. Through these groups you will develop friendships and contacts that may have positive benefits for you. The more social support you have, the more likely you are to stay active and engaged: an outcome that leads to better functioning and slower disease progression.

Health benefits

Non-medication treatments may have benefits for your physical health as well as your mental health. By staying active, maintaining your physical fitness, and increasing you social contacts, you may be better able to manage your other chronic illnesses. Exercise, for example, decreases the risk of cardiovascular and respiratory disease while improving your muscle strength. Exercise and movement therapies, such as dance therapy or yoga, can also decrease your risk of falls. People with progressive memory loss are at a higher risk of falls as they progress in their disease. Non-medication treatments may actually decrease your chances of falling later on by increasing your strength and balance. Engaging in these non-medication treatments that focus on wellness and maintaining your health makes a lot of sense. The sooner you start wellness-focussed treatments, the more likely you are to have positive benefits for your mental and physical functioning.

Scientific support for non-medication treatments

You probably understand that a great deal of research has gone into the development of medications for progressive memory loss. What might surprise you is that a great deal of research has also been done on non-medication treatments and activities for people with progressive memory loss. I will not go into detail, but it may be helpful for you to understand why non-medication treatments may have a positive impact on your disease process. Studies done mostly with animals have shown that if the animal is put into a setting or environment that is enriched, the animal will have a better chance of maintaining mental ability. In other words, just being in an environment with a lot of activities and stimulation, an enriched environment, allows the brain to develop new nerve cells. This enriched environment can also help maintain the function of existing nerve cells, even cells that are damaged. When similar studies were done with humans with some type of brain injury, the same results were found in the human brain. People with severe head injuries, usually from automobile accidents, who were stimulated with a lot of different types of activities, regained some of the brain functions that were lost because of the brain injury. These studies do *not* suggest that different types of brain stimulation are a cure for damage to the brain. These studies do suggest, however, that different types of stimulation may have positive benefits for protecting the nerve cells in the brain. These studies also suggest that, as nerve cells are damaged, other cells may be able to take over the function of the damaged cells if they receive the proper type of stimulation. These studies help to understand why non-medication treatments might help slow the loss of memory and help preserve mental functioning.

What to expect

What might you expect, then, from taking part in non-medication treatment and activities? The results will vary from one person to another. Often we think when we take part in any kind of treatment, including medications, that we will improve our mental functioning. We expect that we are actually going to get better. Improving your mental functioning is one possible outcome. You may see improvement both from medications and non-medication treatments. You are more likely to see improvements from a combination of both types of treatments. With a diagnosis of dementia or progressive memory loss, however, a positive effect of non-medication treatments can be just maintaining your function. With any disease that is progressive in nature, maintaining your function is a positive outcome. So, you may not always see improvement or better functioning, but you may maintain your mental functioning longer by taking part in non-medication treatments. A third positive outcome may be the slowing of the loss of memory. Again, with any illness that is progressive, if the progression of loss can be slowed, that is also a positive outcome. Non-medication treatments may result in any of these three possible outcomes for you. At the very best, you may see improvement in your mental functioning. You may have improved physical and mental ability if you participate in exercise or activity-based treatments. Treatments designed to stimulate mental functioning may help you maintain your mental ability for a longer period of time. All of these possible outcomes are well worth the time and energy you will invest in non-medication treatments.

The following stories are true examples of two people who have very different approaches to managing their memory loss. Morris's story is a great example of someone who embraced non-medication treatments to help him keep his mental abilities as long as possible. The second story is about Pam, a person who decided there was little she could do for herself. The outcomes from both stories are quite different.

Morris's story

Morris was an intelligent, interesting, and active retired professor in his early eighties. When diagnosed with Alzheimer's disease, Morris left his home and moved to a totally different part of the country to be closer to his family. For many people, this move and loss of old friends would have been depressing and resulted in social isolation. Morris, however, took exactly the opposite approach. He decided that instead of giving in to his diagnosis he was going to take positive action. Morris decided he would do all he could to stay healthy and mentally active. Being a scientist all of his life, one of the first things Morris did was read and learn as much as he could about his disease. He then talked with his physician about which treatments were best for him. He learned about his medications and what to expect from them. And, he talked with his physician and family about other non-medication treatments that might also help. Morris then chose treatments that went along with his personality, lifestyle, and interests. He joined an exercise group, but not a typical exercise group. Instead, Morris joined a group that did tai chi exercises. This exercise form focuses on strength, balance, and relaxation, and it matched Morris's interest exactly. Morris also took part in swimming exercises, as he had always enjoyed being near and in water.

In addition to the exercise treatments, Morris found non-medication activities that stimulated his mental processes. As he had been a teacher as well as a scientist, Morris began tutoring his housekeeper, who was studying chemistry—a topic that he knew well. This tutoring activity fit well with Morris's desire to teach and provided mental exercises for Morris. Morris found mental exercises both on the computer and in books to further stimulate his mind. He continued to read the literature in his field. Morris also learned how to use different computer programs than he had never used before. Using his computer was not only something he enjoyed, but it gave Morris a different type of mental stimulation. All of these non-medication activities helped Morris retain his mental abilities and buffer the effects of his disease.

As Morris was a widower, he took steps to become more socially active. Through his synagogue, he met a lovely woman and actually began dating in his early eighties. With her, he went to movies, concerts, plays, and any cultural event that fitted his interests. In a given week, Morris might attend four to five different activities in the community, all of which he enjoyed. Throughout his early memory loss, these different types of social and recreational activities helped Morris function at his highest level. He also took part in many lectures or learning activities that taught him more about his disease and how to manage its effects.

The combination of exercise, mental stimulation, and social and recreational activities helped Morris to maintain his mental abilities. Morris stayed in his own home much longer than he might have had he not taken part in so many non-medication treatments. Morris was in many ways an exceptional individual. However, many people may have these same benefits if they follow Morris's example.

Pam's story

Pam's response to her diagnosis was very different from Morris' response. Pam was in her mid-seventies when she was diagnosed with Alzheimer's disease. She had lived alone and had been widowed for a number of years. During her adult years she spent most of her time working to provide for her two daughters. When Pam learned of her diagnosis, the first thing she did was to give up her apartment and move into an assisted living facility. With this move, in many ways, Pam decided that because of her diagnosis she would no longer try to stay physically fit. She was strong and capable and could have done almost any type of physical activity. Instead, Pam just spent most of her time sitting in her small apartment watching television. Even though exercise programs were available in the facility, Pam refused to attend. She also refused to attend most of the social and mentally stimulating activities that took place. In addition to watching television, Pam waited for her daughter to visit. Because she was bored and refused to take part in activities, she was often unkind to her daughter when she did visit. Yet, Pam longed for more time with her daughter. Pam also started to dwell on her past. She regretted some things she had done or not done previously in her life. Pam eventually became depressed as she was not able to think about her future in any positive way. As Pam refused to take part in any of the non-medication treatments that were available to her, she declined in her mental abilities much faster than she might have had she chosen to be more active. She also felt as if she had no control over her disease. Pam continued to be lonely and depressed throughout her later years.

Non-medication treatments and activities

A variety of non-medication treatments and activities have been tested for people with progressive memory loss. Many of these treatments are available no matter where you live. The types of treatments that are available may vary from one country to another, however. All of the non-medication treatments have some benefits for mental functioning. How do you choose what treatments and activities are best for you? First, you might want to think about what treatment or activity you would enjoy the most. You may have enjoyed some of the treatments in the past or found them interesting. You are more likely to stay with and learn an activity that fits with your personality and your interests. For instance, if you have never enjoyed dancing, then dance-related treatments would not be the best choice. However, if you have always been interested in writing but have never really taken the time to write, now might be the best time to join a creative writing group. A new and interesting activity may stimulate your brain in different ways. But, you also want the activity to be enjoyable. Remember, you are more likely to continue an activity that you find rewarding and positive.

Second, you are most likely to be successful in a treatment or activity that fits with your strengths. With progressive memory loss, the abilities that remain the strongest are those that you have used throughout your life. If you played an instrument much of your life, then activities that have to do with music or playing your instrument might be the activities you will be most successful at doing. If you have always enjoyed puzzles or games, then card groups or word puzzles might be your most successful activities. Fitting the treatments and activities to your previous strengths is another way to design a treatment program that will work for you.

Exercise

Exercise treatments and activities have many benefits for both the mind and body. Studies of exercise treatments have consistently found benefits for people with memory loss, including improved mental ability. The types of exercise treatments available will vary from community to community. However, some types of exercise programs are more common than others. Walking programs as a form of exercise are commonly offered in a variety of settings. Walking programs generally use individual guidelines for walking, based on your physical ability. Walking exercises can help stimulate you mentally while building strength and endurance, especially lower leg strength. Other common types of exercise treatments include strength-building exercises, such as weight-lifting or using large bands to increase resistance and strength. Both walking and strength-building exercise programs have been developed specifically for people with memory loss. Swimming is another exercise that is common for older adults. Swimming exercises have the benefit of being non-weightbearing, making it easy for people with arthritic joints or muscle disorders. Swimming exercises are generally well-supervised, making swimming a safe and enjoyable form of exercise.

Some non-traditional exercises, such as tai chi and yoga, have benefits for muscle strength and balance. Also, both tai chi and yoga require that you concentrate when doing the exercise. In other words, tai chi and yoga cannot be done mindlessly. You can walk and do strength-building exercises while thinking of other things—you do not need to focus on the exercise to do it successfully. But, you must focus your attention on your body movements when doing tai chi and yoga. Because you must pay attention to the movements, both tai chi and yoga may have greater benefits for your mental functioning compared to other exercise forms. Tai chi and yoga also involve slow, purposeful body movements. The slow movements are particularly appealing to older adults. Slow movements also allow for the extra time it takes to process information for people with progressive memory loss. As the movements involve shifting of your body weight, both tai chi and yoga can help develop and sustain balance—a benefit that might prevent falls. Tai chi and yoga also have relaxation as part of the exercise. Relaxation can also help decrease stress and focus your attention. Lower stress can also help with your memory and thinking ability.

Whatever type of exercise you choose, you should fit the exercise to your own interests. Most exercises are done in a classroom, usually with about 10–15 people. Most groups meet two to three times a week. Once you have learned the exercises, you can do them in the comfort of your home. Exercise is a good activity to do with your spouse or family member. You are more likely to enjoy the exercises if you do them with someone who enjoys them as well. The

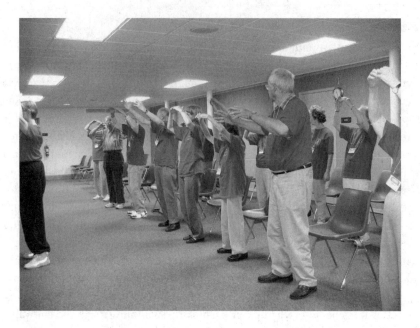

positive effects of the exercise depend on the exercise form, the amount of exercise, and the length of time in which you participate. You can expect some positive benefits of exercise on your physical and mental functioning, however, no matter which type of exercise treatment you choose. Once you stop exercising, however, the positive effects of exercising start to decline within a few months of stopping. You must continue with exercises, then, to constantly have the benefits. So, starting and staying with an exercise treatment now can be important for your future functioning and quality of life.

Mental stimulation

Mental exercises are designed to directly stimulate your thinking and your brain. These exercises include mental training and stimulation programs. Mental training programs are designed to help with memory, attention, and problem-solving. Mental training programs can also help with other areas, such as activities of daily living like shopping, household tasks, and financial management. Mental training programs use two basic approaches to help with mental functioning. One approach is to help you compensate for the areas of mental functioning where you have difficulty. Tasks that may help compensate for losses include asking questions during learning, focussing on one task at a time, or learning by using your senses such as hearing, smell, and touch. Mental training programs use aids such as memory notebooks, visual cues, and calendars to help with memory and functioning. Memory can also be improved

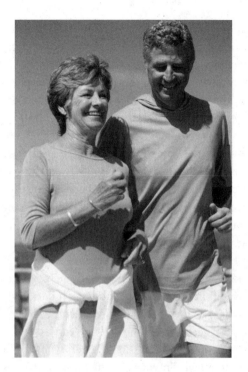

through practice, pairing a word with a picture, and repeated recall of information over time.

Mental stimulation treatments can also benefit memory and mental functioning. Mental stimulation treatments can be active or passive. Active treatments include things such as group discussions of current events, solving a puzzle, or word games. Passive mental stimulation treatments may include listening to a poetry reading, watching a play, or listening to music. Mental stimulation treatments are available in a group setting, on computers, and in printed form. For example, one book called *Don't Forget: Easy Exercises for a Better Memory* (Lapp, 1995) includes a variety of different exercises designed to stimulate your thinking and your memory. This type of printed guide allows you to select the mental exercises that you would enjoy the most and that you would be willing to do on a regular basis. Doing mental stimulation exercises in a group may be helpful, as you would be learning with others. In a group setting, you will benefit from the support of group members while you are learning. The group support may lessen any frustration you might have when learning new tasks and information. These groups are often called "cognitive stimulation" groups. You may find it harder to locate a cognitive stimulation group in your area than a support group. You can ask your primary healthcare provider if they know of a cognitive stimulation group in your area. You can learn about these groups through any type of local Alzheimer's Association or other group that focusses on people with memory loss.

Computer programs have been developed that have mental exercises to stimulate your memory and thinking. Online groups and programs are available that also allow you to interact with others as you do the programs. Other computers programs have crossword puzzles or word games that you can do on your own. One advantage of computer programs and online groups is that they keep you connected to the outside world while stimulating your brain. Computer programs are available 24 hours a day. They can be done in the home or your computer can travel with you. For people who are comfortable using a computer, computer-based programs can be a valuable source of mental stimulation and learning.

The positive benefits of mental stimulation programs include improved memory and thinking, fewer mistakes, better judgment, improved self-care, less depression, and overall improved mental ability. Studies have found that these positive effects can last after you stop the treatment. Positive effects on mental functioning have been seen for as long as two years after the treatment's end. Because of these immediate and long-term benefits, you will want to include a mental stimulation treatment in your non-medication treatment program.

Life review and reminiscence therapy

Other mental stimulation activities include reminiscence therapy and life reviews. Both activities are generally done in a group setting. These activities can also be done with family members or friends. Healthcare providers such as social workers, occupational therapists, or recreational therapists often conduct the reminiscence and life review therapies. Life review and reminiscence therapies involve recording and discussing your life in relation to today. You are encouraged to recall the positive times in your life. You may also want to write about or record past events for other family members. You may do other activities such as talk about or arrange photographs to help remind you of your past. Long-term memory is used in life review therapy. Long-term memory is the recall of events that happened earlier in your life, when you were a child or young adult. Long-term memory is often preserved with memory loss, although your memory about recent events is impaired. Therapies that focus on the distant past can stimulate your brain and allow you to use your long-term memory. Recalling the past and thinking of how your past relates to the present can help you stay in touch with who you are as a person. Life reviews help you to recall times in your past that were meaningful. If these therapies are available in your community, taking part in a life review or reminiscence group could be positive for you.

Social and creative programs

Non-medication treatments that involve social and creative activities take many forms and are widely available. The activities draw upon the interests and abilities of people with progressive memory loss. The activities are also designed to help maintain or improve mental functioning. Social and creative activity programs can include diverse activities such as card playing, dancing, creative writing, and art or drawing projects. Creative activities can also include recreational events, such as art shows and garden walks. These social and creative activities, such as dance therapy, allow you to be with the same people over time. Taking part in these programs with other people with progressive memory loss may ease any discomfort you might have about trying something new. Writing programs have also been developed for people with progressive memory loss. The writing programs help individuals with progressive memory loss by stimulating creative thinking. Using words also stimulates specific parts of the brain affected by diseases that cause memory loss. Writing programs give the person the option of writing poems, short stories, or other creative works. The writing activity alone is stimulating and often rewarding. College courses just for people with progressive memory loss have also been developed. These courses are designed to teach self-care and healthy activities to maintain function. The college courses also give people with progressive memory loss the chance to be in a stimulating environment.

With all these choices, you can select the social and creative activities that are best for you. For example, you may be interested in writing activities, but do not enjoy going to art exhibits. Different agencies offer different types of social and creative programs. Social and recreational activities are often offered by local recreation or park groups. You can also find them through service centers for older adults in your local community. These social and creative programs may also be offered through adult day care centers. If the program is designed for people with memory loss, the activity is often led by a healthcare professional. Social and creative activities stimulate your brain in ways that are different from other activities. These programs also tend to be enjoyed by people with progressive memory loss. The combined benefits of enjoyment and mental stimulation make these activities well worth including in your non-medication treatment program.

Companion programs

Companion programs have been developed for people with progressive memory loss to help them interact with others, including animals, in a very purposeful way. Human companion programs often match a person with memory loss with a volunteer with similar interests. The volunteer can be an older adult, college student, or any person with similar interests to you. Interacting with a volunteer can stimulate your thinking by the activities you do together and just by talking together about meaningful events. Activities may include things such as outdoor walks, dining, or going to community events. Volunteer companions give you support outside of your family. Trusting and enjoyable relationships are often formed with volunteer companions.

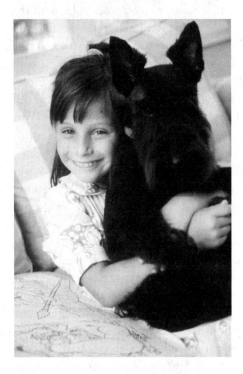

Pet companion programs are also available in communities around the world. Pet companion programs use trained pets, often domestic animals such as cats and dogs, to provide comfort to people with progressive memory loss. Pet companions are non-threatening and offer affection. If you have enjoyed pets in the past, a pet companion can keep you from being lonely. If you try a pet companion and find it to be positive, you may decide that having a pet of your own is best. Both of these companion programs can take place in or outside the home.

If you are more comfortable in your own home, companion programs provide a mentally stimulating activity where you are most comfortable. If you take part in a companion program outside your home, you will stimulate your memory and thinking in different ways. Companion programs are not for everyone. If you are the type of person that would enjoy a companion, these programs can meet some of your social needs while having positive effects on memory and mental ability.

Sensory stimulation

Some non-medication treatments use your senses, such as smell, touch, and hearing, to stimulate thinking and memory. These treatments are called sensory stimulation activities. For example, aroma therapy uses candles and other sources of pleasant aromas to both stimulate your sense of smell and provide relaxation. Music therapy uses music that you find pleasant. The music is generally played at times when you can benefit from both mental stimulation and relaxation. Often music is played in late morning or afternoon to help you relax before mealtimes. Sensory stimulation can take the form of using interesting colors, paintings, or fabrics in your home. Varying textures and visual objects can activate your thinking and interest. Sensory stimulation activities are easy to use in your home. In addition to activating your memory and thinking, sensory stimulation activities are pleasant and can provide comfort.

Technology support programs

Some non-medication activities use technology to enhance thinking and memory. Technology programs also help people with progressive memory loss to stay in their homes. For example, computers can be placed in the home to remind you of your schedule, to remind you to take your medications, or to monitor your activity. These computers can be linked to family members that live in another location. Your family member can communicate with you through the computer and update your schedule each day from a distance. Another support program is designed to teach people with memory loss how to use cell phones. This program can help you use a cell phone wherever you are, which allows you to be more comfortable away from home. With memory loss, you may forget how to get from one place to another, even if you have used the same route for many years. With a cell phone, you can contact someone if you are unsure of finding your way. Learning to use a cell phone increases your safety. Global positioning systems (GPS) are more expensive than cell phones, but can also be used to help you stay safe. A GPS system can be placed in an automobile. The GPS system will give you directions from one location to another, without distracting you from driving. Electronic monitoring systems have also been tested in the homes of people with memory loss. The monitoring system uses cameras to track your movements. The system alerts family members or other people watching the monitor about any unsafe activities. Home monitoring systems may feel like an invasion of your privacy, however. You should discuss the benefits and costs of any of these technology support programs before investing in them. Some technology support programs can stimulate your thinking, such as learning to use cell phones and computers, and can also help you stay independent.

Support groups and cognitive therapies

Two other non-medication treatments are support groups and cognitive therapies. Both of these treatments were described in previous chapters, so they will not be described here. Non-medication treatments that combine different activities may have the greatest benefits for memory and thinking. For example, support groups can be combined with cognitive therapies or exercise. The results of combined activities are often stronger and more positive as the brain is stimulated in different ways.

Other activities may help your mental functioning, but have not been tested through research. These activities are included as they might be positive for you.

Travel

Travel is also an activity that can stimulate the brain in a number of different ways. Memory loss doesn't mean you have to stop traveling. Although people with progressive memory loss may become more confused and forgetful when away from home, planning for a trip can help prevent some negative outcomes. Traveling can be positive for you without taking long, costly trips. Travel can mean going to another community for a special event. You may travel to visit a friend or relative that you enjoy being with. You can travel safely through travel groups or by traveling with trusted friends and family members. Planning can also help you travel safely. You want to plan for adequate rest. So, make sure that the schedule is not too demanding. If you are tired or lack sleep, you are more likely to have more trouble with your memory and thinking. It may also be best to travel in small groups to lessen the confusion. Keeping your daily schedule as close to your usual schedule will be helpful. For example, you will want to go to bed and get up around the same time as you did at home. You will want to keep mealtimes the same as your home schedule. With planning, you can travel safely while stimulating your brain and thinking.

Spiritual care

Memory loss does not change a person's spiritual or religious beliefs. In fact, the diagnosis of progressive memory loss may make the need for spiritual care even greater. People with progressive memory loss still recall prayers or hymns that they have enjoyed throughout their lives. Even when names are forgotten, you may still have a sense of the presence of a higher being. After working with people with memory loss, one pastor observed that even when the brain fails, "God is known in the human heart." People with progressive memory loss may continue to benefit from taking part in religious activities, especially if religion has been important in the past. Prayers, hymns, communion, and religious meals and rituals can be reassuring. Meeting your spiritual needs can help you stay in touch with who you are as a person. Not all religious leaders, such as ministers, priests, and rabbis, understand that people with progressive memory loss may benefit from their care. You may need to ask your spiritual leader for personal visits or support, if needed. Taking care of your spiritual needs can have benefits for both your thinking and sense of personhood.

Building a treatment program

What type of non-medication treatment program do you want to build for yourself? While thinking about a treatment program, you will want to include different types of treatments and activities. Different activities will stimulate the brain in different ways. So, a combination of activities may produce the best results for you. A powerful treatment program might include some form of exercise, a mental stimulation activity, a creative activity, and some type of social activity. If you are interested in the arts or artistic expression, you will want to add some kind of art-based program. An art-based program does not have to be painting or drawing. Instead it could be a reading group, writing program, or an art appreciation class. Including a variety of treatments and activities allows you to express yourself in different ways while benefiting your body and brain. The personal journal found at the end of this chapter can be used to outline your non-medication treatment program.

✓

YOUR NON-MEDICATION TREATMENT JOURNAL

Treatment	Steps to start treatment	Interests/ability
1.	1.	
	2.	
	3.	
	4.	
	5.	
2.	1.	
	2.	
	3.	
	4.	
	5.	
3.	1.	
	2.	
	3.	
	4.	
	5.	
4.	1.	
	2.	
	3.	
	4.	
	5.	
5.	1.	
	2.	
	3.	
	4.	
	5.	

COMMON NON-MEDICATION TREATMENTS (1)

- Exercise programs:
  - walking
  - swimming
  - strength and resistance training
  - tai chi
  - yoga
- Mental stimulation
- Life review and reminiscence
- Social and creative programs:
  - card groups
  - creative writing
  - recreational activities: art shows and garden walks
  - dance therapy
  - art therapy
  - social activities: dinner, plays, cultural events
- Companion programs:
  - human
  - pet

COMMON NON-MEDICATION TREATMENTS (2)

- Sensory stimulation:
  - aroma therapy
  - music therapy
  - varying textures and visual objects
- Technology support:
  - in-home computers
  - electronic monitoring systems
  - cell phones
  - global positioning systems
- Support groups
- Cognitive therapies
- Travel
- Spiritual care

CHAPTER 9

Finding Hope

One of the first responses following a diagnosis of progressive memory loss is to hope for a magic pill. Putting all of your hope for the future on an easy cure or fix can be one way to avoid dealing with the diagnosis. In today's medical environment of miracle cures, the thought of a magic pill to cure or fix the progressive memory loss is very appealing. Once you get past the need to find the magic pill or realize that is not the only path to finding hope, you can start to adjust to the diagnosis. The first thing is to acknowledge or become aware of changes within you. With awareness of these changes, you will begin to find ways to protect yourself. You will be more aware of your strengths and the areas where you are vulnerable. You will also start to monitor how the changes affect the way you view yourself and the way others view you: your perception of yourself changes very slowly, even with changes in ability. However, over time, you will have new expectations of yourself. With these new expectations, you can then positively set about constructing your life to fit your abilities. All of these steps are part of adjusting to progressive memory loss. The outcomes of this adjustment are much more active and positive than waiting for the discovery of the magic pill.

Finding hope is one response that helps you adjust to the diagnosis. First of all, it can help you cope with the changes that you are experiencing. We know from research that having hope actually helps with healing and possibly even with survival. The other positive part of having hope is that it gives you some control over your diagnosis. By having hope and being more active, you are not putting yourself in a position of just "being done to." Instead, you are in a position of having some active control over your disease. Experiencing hope gives you the incentive to stay active and engaged. Hope allows you to adjust to the diagnosis of progressive memory loss in ways that are more positive for you and those around you.

In addition to helping adjust to the diagnosis, hope obviously allows you to have a much more positive outlook and attitude. People who live with hope are generally more open to and accepting of what their future may hold. People who live with hope also have an overall higher quality of life. Although you might not be able to directly change what is happening inside your brain, you certainly can influence your quality of life. Having a hopeful outlook is one way to improve your quality of life. People who are hopeful are also more comfortable, not only with themselves, but with the people around them. The comfort you gain from having hope can help you be more relaxed and positive when you interact with others. When you think about the types of people you want to be around, you most generally want to be around people who are positive. People are often more positive because they live with hope. Your friends and family members will feel the same way. Having hope allows you to be more positive with friends and family members, resulting in better relationships.

How hope is experienced

At first, you may think that hope is not possible—not with a diagnosis of progressive memory loss. But, hope is possible and can be experienced in different ways. First, hope is experienced inwardly, affecting all that you do and think. Inward experiences of hope affect your general attitude toward life, including your diagnosis. People who are hopeful are often the people who "fight the good fight." People who live with hope do not have a defeatist attitude, but have an attitude of being in control of their destiny. Inward hope allows you to mobilize your resources and actively find ways to manage your memory loss.

You may find yourself hoping for different things after your diagnosis. Before, your inward hopes may have been long-reaching. You may have hoped for events or life changes years in advance. For example, before your diagnosis you may have hoped for long vacations, new challenges, or new ways to earn income after retirement. With memory loss, hope is often limited to a shorter time period. You may find yourself now hoping for a good day or a happy meal with your family. Your hope may extend to just the next day or two, rather than months or years in advance. Focussing your hope on a shorter timespan helps keep your hope alive. You may try saying to yourself every morning, "What can I hope for today?"

Hope is also experienced outwardly. People with hope are more likely to not be seen as just a score on a memory test or a person with dementia. The person who lives with hope is more likely to have an outward expression of him or herself. Your outward expressions of hope identify who you are and how you live. It is helpful to know that scores on a memory test do not directly relate to your quality of life, wellbeing, or how your memory loss affects your daily life. What does directly affect your quality of life is how you live with the diagnosis, including your outward expressions of hope.

Examples of living with hope

Living with hope alone can make a tremendous difference in every aspect of living with progressive memory loss. In the first story, you will learn about a person who should have much more despair than hope. However, the person in the first story, Michelle, actually has a much higher quality of life and a more positive experience with memory loss because she has hope. The second example on the next page is the story of a woman, Helen, who lost hope when she was diagnosed with progressive memory loss. Her life became filled with despair, although just changing her attitude and finding hope would have allowed her to have a much higher quality of life. In both stories, the effects of the memory loss on each person are very much the same. Having or not having hope makes the difference in the outcomes for both people.

Michelle's story

Michelle was very young when she was diagnosed with progressive memory loss. She was in her mid-fifties. She knew that the diagnosis meant that she would experiences changes more quickly than someone who was older. Michelle, because of her young age, had much more to lose than many people who are diagnosed later in life. Michelle's husband had an active career. She was a young grandmother with very young grandchildren and a growing family. Despite having so much to lose, Michelle was filled with hope for the future. She approached her diagnosis in a very positive way. She increased the amount of exercising she was doing, priding herself on outpacing her husband during their evening runs. She talked about and continued to enjoy her grandchildren a great deal. She carried photographs of her grandchildren with her. When it became difficult for her to find words, she would use the photographs to express herself. She continued to be a very social person. She attended support programs, not only at her church, but also in the community. She knew how important it was to have support and to have positive interactions with others. Michelle rarely felt sorry for herself, and was a joy to be around. Michelle also participated in research studies to help fight her disease. And, although she would love to find the magic pill, she did not put her life on hold and wait for it. She continued doing all she actively could do to fight the good fight, and enjoy life to the greatest extent possible while living with progressive memory loss. Despite her young age and the severity of her disease, Michelle's hope allowed her to have a high quality of life.

Helen's story

Helen's story is quite different. Helen was diagnosed with progressive memory loss in her late seventies, at a time when she was a widow living alone in a small community where she had lived most of her adult life. Shortly after her diagnosis, Helen became very distraught. With every new challenge and every loss, Helen would become more and more discouraged. She quickly gave in to the effects of progressive memory loss, giving up her home at a time when she was still able to manage to live by herself. Helen's first move was into an assisted living facility where she, for a while, enjoyed the company of her daughter. Because of her negative attitudes and her fear of embarrassment, she spent much of her time in her room in her apartment. Because of this isolation, Helen did not interact with other people at the facility. Helen's negative attitude and despair made it difficult for her family members to spend a great deal of time with her, especially her younger grandchildren. Whenever I visited Helen, she always became tearful and emotionally upset about her diagnosis. Her general outlook was one of defeat. She had lost her home, although she chose to give it up and she had moved from the community she loved. Helen could think only of her losses and not on the positive aspects of her life. Because of this, Helen spent much of her time in despair. Helen lost her ability to enjoy the time she had with her daughter and grandchildren. Helen's loss of hope resulted in a much lower quality of life even though she had the ability to enjoy others and do many things she had done in the past.

Where to find hope
Hope through contributing to others

So where can you find hope with a diagnosis of progressive memory loss? Hope can be found in many areas of your life. First of all, hope can be found in the successes that you experience every single day. Just being able to contribute in a positive way to the lives of others adds to your own wellbeing and hope for the future. As you are able to give positively to others, including family members and friends, you can be hopeful about continuing to contribute to their wellbeing and your own. For instance, you may not feel comfortable driving your grandchildren to activities or watching them by yourself. This does not mean, however, that you will stop being a positive person in their lives. Through simple activities, such as attending their school functions or sporting events, you can remain a positive part of their lives. One man in my support group describes the positive effects he has on his family in a beautiful way. He says that he knows how much he means to his grandchildren when he sees the big smiles on their faces when they visit. Just continuing to be "grandpa" gives him hope for the future as he knows he will continue to be an important part of their lives. Hope can be found in the simple enjoyment of being with someone who is important to you—and knowing you are important to them.

Hope through success

Hope can be found in the successes you have with everyday problem-solving. Although progressive memory loss presents you with new challenges, it also provides opportunities for success. Hope can be found in just doing something well. For example, you may find that you can still prepare your favorite dish or dessert for family gatherings, if you just write the recipe in simple, one-step directions. Problem-solving to continue doing this activity and to make it successful can give you hope that you can continue the activity in the weeks and months ahead. Any activity that provides you with enjoyment and can still be done well can provide you with hope. Enjoying simple successes not only gives you hope for your own quality of life, but hope that you can continue to contribute to the lives of others.

Hope through watching others succeed

Hope can come from the feedback that you get from the people and groups with whom you spend time. If you are part of a support group, you can find hope in seeing other people in the group do well. Often, in a support group, you will be able to look around the group and see others who are managing their memory loss in very positive ways. Watching others have positive outcomes can give you hope for your own success. Hope can be found in the understanding that you have of other people with progressive memory loss. It is often said that no one can really "walk in your shoes." While you may not be able to fully understand another's experience, you will be able to come closer to that understanding because of your own experience with memory loss. So, the hope that you find in seeing the positive ways that others manage their memory loss will increase your hope for your own future.

Hope through not being alone

Hope can be found in the time that you spend with those you love. Continuing to be trusted and accepted by those you love the most will give you hope for the future. Often, time with family becomes more valuable after you have a diagnosis of progressive memory loss. You can find hope in the fact that you will not need to face memory loss alone. You will know that your family will always be with you and be part of the journey. Many people in my support groups have told me that their relationship with their husband or wife actually became stronger after they were diagnosed with progressive memory loss. Your relationship with your spouse may become closer because both of you will be managing or dealing with the same issues. Memory loss often brings out the kinder or more loving parts of the person and their spouse. The quality and quantity of positive times with your family and spouse can give you hope through knowing that you will not be facing your memory loss alone.

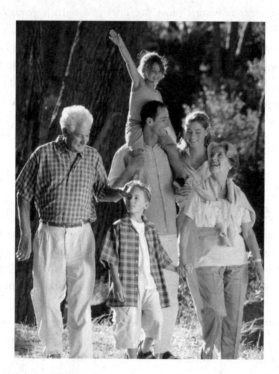

Hope through faith

Hope can be found by keeping in touch with those parts of you that remain very much alive and intact. Often, people who have had a strong spiritual or religious belief in the past continue to find comfort and hope in that spiritual awareness within them. Even as memory loss becomes more severe, you will still be able to recall the prayers and hymns that you have read or sung all of your life. You will still be able to find comfort in those prayers and hymns. You will be able to find comfort and peace in the connections to a higher being that you have found throughout your life. This spiritual or religious connection can give you the hope that you are not alone, but that a higher being is with you in your memory loss, helping you along the way.

Hope through feeling

Your emotional ties to others will remain alive and real for you, even as memory loss becomes more severe. You will always be able to experience the "loves of your life." I saw this most clearly in a woman, Carol, diagnosed with progressive memory loss in her late sixties. She had been married for many years, but had always centered her life on her husband. As her memory loss progressed, it became more and more difficult for Carol to be with her husband and his activities. She eventually lost her ability to communicate with her husband through words. She did find ways, however, to connect with her husband in very loving ways. When he would bend to kiss her as he was preparing to leave, she would often pull him near or hold on to his hand. It was obvious that Carol found comfort in that close, physical contact. This ability to continue to experience true love and connections with others is a source of hope for the future, despite memory loss.

Hope through progress

Hope can be found in a changing culture. At one point, a diagnosis of progressive memory loss resulted in negative responses by healthcare professionals and society at large. Although a diagnosis of memory loss often results in stigma and unnecessarily negative interactions, society is becoming more sensitive to the individual with progressive memory loss. Some highly respected healthcare professionals have written wonderful and sensitive books and articles about the need to be aware of supporting the person with progressive memory loss. As well-known people, such as Ronald Reagan, a United States President, announce that they have progressive memory loss, people in general are becoming more accepting of the diagnosis. The diagnosis of dementia is no longer being whispered about in back rooms and behind closed doors. Like cancer and HIV/AIDS, progressive memory loss is becoming more of a household word—resulting in less fear of the unknown. These changing values and increasing acceptance should result in more positive responses from others and greater support as you face your diagnosis.

The magic pill is not available at this time. However, new treatments for progressive memory loss provide some hope for more aggressive therapies in the future. Although a cure for dementia is still eluding researchers, some medications and vaccines that are currently being tested are promising. Vaccines have the potential to interfere with the disease process in Alzheimer's disease, allowing for a slowing of nerve cell loss and damage. Other medications that are being tested may also interfere with the disease process. These medications may help stop substances, such as plaque, from forming on nerve cells or help remove the substance once it is formed. Both actions can stop or greatly decrease nerve cell loss and damage. A number of other treatments are being tested, including things such as electrical stimulation, altering the amount of cerebrospinal fluid in the brain, and use of other drugs such as antioxidants and cholesterol-lowering drugs. Together, these new directions in treatment give hope through the progress that is being made in finding new ways to fight progressive memory loss.

Living with hope

Even with hope, you may have days filled with frustration or sadness. These varying responses are to be expected with any disease that is progressive in nature and affects how you function. Finding and holding on to hope, however, prevents the bleak days from taking over your life. Hope gives you control over how you respond to your disease. Hope allows you to look to the future with promise. Hope changes how you view the potential that each day holds. Hope enriches your time with family and friends. Hope helps you celebrate each success and not be defeated by each failure. Hope lets you continue to celebrate who you are as a person. Hope is worth striving for and keeping in your life.

References

Adams, T. and Gardiner, P. (2005) Communication and interaction within dementia triads: developing a theory for relationship-centred care. *Dementia 4*, (2), 185–205.

Davis, R. and Davis, B. (1989) *My Journey into Alzheimer's Disease.* Wheaton, IL: Tyndale House.

Edwards, H. and Chapman, H. (2004a) Communicating in family aged care dyads Part 1: The influence of stereotypical role expectations. *Quality in Ageing 5* (2), 3–12.

Edwards, H. and Chapman, H. (2004b) Caregiver-care receiver communication Part 2: Overcoming the influence of stereotypical role expectations. *Quality in Ageing 5*, (3), 3–13.

Feil, N. (1993) *The Validation Breakthrough: Simple Techniques for Communicating with People with Alzheimer's Type Dementia.* Baltimore, MD: Health Professionals Press.

Henderson, C. (1998) *Partial View: An Alzheimer's Journal.* Dallas, TX: Southern Methodist University Press.

Kitwood, T. (1997) *Dementia Reconsidered.* Oxford: Oxford University Press.

Kitwood, T. (1997) The experience of dementia. *Aging and Mental Health 1*, 13–22.

Kuhn, D. (2003) *Alzheimer's Early Stages: First Steps for Family, Friends, and Caregivers* (2nd edition). Berkeley, CA: Hunter House, Inc.

Lapp, D.C. (1995) *Don't Forget: Easy Exercises for a Better Memory.* New York, NY: Addison Wesley Publishing.

McGowin, D.F. (1993) *Living in the Labyrinth: A Personal Journey through the Maze of Alzheimer's.* New York, NY: Delacorte Press.

Orange, J.B. and Lubinski, R.B. (1996) Conversational repair by individuals with dementia of the Alzheimer's type. *Journal of Speech and Hearing Research 39*, 881–895.

Small, J.A., Gutman, G., Makela, S. and Hillhouse, B. (2003). Effectiveness of communication strategies used by caregivers of persons with Alzheimer's disease during activities of daily living. *Journal of Speech, Language, and Hearing Research 46*, 353–367.

Snyder, L. (2002) Social and family relationships: establishing and maintaining connections. In P.B. Harris (ed.) *The Person with Alzheimer's Disease: Pathways to Understanding the Experience.* Baltimore, MD: The Johns Hopkins Press.

Teri, L. and Gallagher-Thompson, D. (1991) Cognitive-behavioral interventions for treatment of depression in Alzheimer's patients. *The Gerontologist 31*, (3), 413–416.

Bibliography

Adlard, A.P., Perreau, V.M., Pop, V. and Cotman, C.W. (2004) Voluntary exercise decreases amyloid load in a transgenic model of Alzheimer's disease. *Journal of Neuroscience 25*, (17), 4217–4221.

Alzheimer's Disease Progress Report (2000) Bethesda, MD: National Institutes of Health, National Institute on Aging, Alzheimer's Disease Advisory Panel.

Alzheimer Society of Canada (2006) *Engaging People with Early Stage Alzheimer's Disease in the Work of the Alzheimer Society: A Research Report.* www.alzheimer.ca/english/disease/whatsit-intro.htm (accessed August 25 2006).

Arkin, S.M. (1996) Volunteers in partnership: an Alzheimer's rehabilitation program delivered by students. *American Journal of Alzheimer's Disease 11*, 12–22.

Bach-y-Rita, P. (2003) Theoretical basis for brain plasticity after TBI. *Brain Injury 17*, 643–651.

Bach-y-Rita, P. (2003) Late postacute neurologic rehabilitation: neuroscience, engineering, and clinical programs. *Archives of Physical Medicine and Rehabilitation 84*, 1100–1108.

Baker, F.M., Wiley, C., Kokmen, E., Chandra, V. and Schoenberg, B.S. (1999) Delirium episodes during the course of clinically diagnosed Alzheimer's disease. *Journal of the National Medical Association 91*, 625–630.

Benbow, S.M., and Reynolds, D. (2000) Challenging the stigma of Alzheimer's disease. *Hospital Medicine 61*, (3), 174–177.

Brashear, A., Unverzagt, F.W., Kuhn, E.R., Glazier, B.S., Farlow, M.R., Perkins, A.J and Hui, S.L. (1998). Impaired traffic sign recognition in drivers with dementia. *American Journal of Alzheimer's Disease 13*, 131–137.

Brod, M., Stewart, A.L. and Sands, L. (2000) Conceptualization of quality of life in dementia. In S.M. Albert and R.G. Logsdon (eds), *Assessing Quality of Life in Alzheimer's Disease.* New York, NY: Springer Publishing Co.

Brown, L.B., Ott, B.R., Papandonatos, G.D., Sui, Y., Ready, R.E. and Morris, J.C. (2005) Prediction of on-road driving performance in patients with early Alzheimer's disease. *Journal of the American Geriatrics Society 53*, (1), 94–98.

Buettner, L.L. (2006) Peace of mind: a pilot community-based program for older adults with memory loss. *American Journal of Recreation Therapy 13*, (2), 1–7.

Buettner, L.L. and Fitzsimmons, S. (2006) Recreation clubs: an outcome-based alternative to daycare for older adults with memory loss. *Activities Directors' Quarterly for Alzheimer's and Other Dementia Patients 7*, (2), 10–20.

Burgener, S.C. (1999) Predicting quality of life in caregivers of Alzheimer's patients: the role of support from and involvement with the religious community. *Journal of Pastoral Care 53*, (4), 433–446.

Burgener, S.C. (1999) Care decisions in irreversible dementia: who speaks for the patient? *Journal of Gerontological Nursing 25*, (8), 53–55.

Burgener, S.C. and Dickerson-Putman, J. (1999) Assessing the patient in the early stages of irreversible dementia: the relevance of patient perspectives. *Journal of Gerontological Nursing 25*, (2), 33–41.

Burgener, S.C. and Twigg, P. (2002) Relationships among caregiver factors and quality of life in care recipients with irreversible dementia. *Journal of Alzheimer's Disease and Related Disorders 16*, (2), 88–102.

Burgener, S.C. and Twigg, P. (2002) Interventions for persons with irreversible dementia. In P. Archbold and B. Stewart (eds) *Annual Review of Nursing Research.* New York, NY: Springer Publishing Co.

Burgener, S.C., Twigg, P. and Popovich, A. (2005) Measuring psychological well being in cognitively impaired persons. *Dementia: The International Journal of Social Research and Practice 4*, (4), 463–485.

Carr, D.B., LaBarge, E., Dunnigan, K. and Storandt, M. (1998) Differentiating drivers with dementia of the Alzhiemer type from healthy older persons with a traffic sign naming test. *Journal of Gerontology: Medical Sciences 53A*, M135–M139.

Castleman, M., Gallagher-Thompson, D. and Naythons, M. (1999) *There's Still a Person in There: The Complete Guide to Treating and Coping with Alzheimer's.* New York, NY: The Berkley Publishing Company.

Clare, L. (2002) We'll fight it as long as we can: coping with the onset of Alzheimer's disease. *Aging & Mental Health 6*, (2), 139–148.

Clare, L. (2003) Managing threats to self: awareness in early stage Alzheimer's disease. *Social Science & Medicine 57*, 1017–1029.

Clare, L., Wilson, B., Carter, G., Roth, I. and Hodges, J. (2004) Awareness in early-stage dementia: relationship to outcome of cognitive rehabilitation intervention. *Journal of Clinical and Experimental Neuropsychology 26*, (2), 215–226.

Cole, M.G., McCusker, J., Bellavance, F., Primeau, F.J., Bailey, R.F., Bonnycastle, M.J., *et al.* (2002) Systematic detection and multidisciplinary care of delirium in older medical inpatients: a randomized trial. *Canadian Medical Association Journal 167*, 753–759.

Colling, K.B. (1999) Passive behaviors in Alzheimer's disease: a descriptive analysis. *American Journal of Alzheimer's Disease 14*, (1), 27–40.

Cotelli, M., Calabria, M. and Zanetti, O. (2006) Cognitive rehabilitation in Alzheimer's disease. *Aging Clinical and Experimental Research 18*, (2), 141–143.

Cox, D.J., Quillian, W.C., Thorndike, F.P., Kovatchev, B.P. and Hanna, G. (1998) Evaluating driving performance of outpatients with Alzheimer disease. *Journal of the American Board of Family Practice 11*, (4), 264–271.

DeVreese L.P., Neri M., Fiorvanti M., Belloi L. and Zanetti O. (2001) Memory rehabilitation in Alzheimer's disease: a review of progress. *International Journal of Geriatric Psychiatry 16*, (8), 794–809.

Diesfieldt, H.F. and Diesfeldt-Groenendijk, H. (1977) Improving cognitive performance in psychogeriatric patients: the influence of physical exercise. *Age and Ageing 6*, (1), 58–64.

Duchek, J.M., Carr, D.B., Hunt, L., Roe, C.M. *et al.* (2003) Longitudinal driving performance in early-stage dementia of the Alzheimer type. *Journal of the American Geriatrics Society 51*, 1499–1501.

Esposito, E., Rotilio, D., Di Matteo, V., Di Giulio, C., Cacchio, M. and Algeri, S. (2002) A review of specific dietary antioxidants and the effects on biochemical mechanisms related to neurodegenerative processes. *Neurobiology of Aging 23*, (5), 719–735.

Farina, E., Mantovani, F., Fioravanti, R., Rotella, G. *et al.* (2006) Efficacy of recreational and occupational activities associated to psychological support in mild to moderate Alzheimer disease: a multicenter controlled study. *Alzheimer's Disease and Associated Disorders 20*, (4), 275–282.

Fick, D., Agostini, J.V. and Inouye, S.K. (2002) Delirium superimposed on dementia: a systematic review. *Journal of the American Geriatric Society 50*, 1723–1732.

Fick, D. and Foreman, M. (2000) Consequences of not recognizing delirium superimposed on dementia in hospitalized elderly individuals. *Journal of Gerontological Nursing 26*, 30–40.

Fick, D., Kolanowski, A., Waller, J.L. and Inouye, S.K. (2005) Delirium superimposed on dementia in a community-living managed care population: a three year retrospective study of prevalence, costs, and utilization. *The Journals of Gerontology, Series B, Psychological Sciences and Social Sciences 60A*, 748–753.

Fitzsimmons, S. and Buettner, L.L. (2003) Health promotion for the mind, body, and spirit: a college course for older adults with dementia. *American Journal of Alzheimer's Disease and Other Dementias 18*, (5), 282–290.

Goldsilver, P.M. and Gruneir, M.R.B. (2001) Early stage dementia group: an innovative model of support for individuals in the early stages of dementia. *American Journal of Alzheimer's Disease and Other Dementias 16*, (2), 109–114.

Gonzalez-Gross, M., Marcos, A and Pietrzik, K. (2001) Nutrition and cognitive impairment in the elderly. *British Journal of Nutrition 86*, (3), 313–321.

Harris, P.B. (2002) *The Person with Alzheimer's Disease: Pathways to Understanding the Experience.* Baltimore, MD: The Johns Hopkins Press.

Harris, P.B. and Sterin, G.J. (1999) Insider's perspective: defining and preserving the self in dementia. *Journal of Mental Health and Aging 5*, 241–256.

Herzog, A.R., Franks, M.M., Marcus, H.R. and Holmberg, D. (1998) Activities and well-being in older age: effects of self concept and educational attainment. *Psychology and Aging 13*, 179–185.

Hoffman M., Hock C. and Muller-Spahn F. (1996) Computer-based cognitive training in Alzheimer's disease patients. *Annals of the New York Academy of Science 17*, 249–254.

Hunter, K.I., Linn, M.W. (1981) Psychosocial differences between elderly volunteers and non-volunteers. *International Journal of Aging and Human Development 12*, 205–213.

Inouye, S.K. (2006) Delirium in older persons. *New England Journal of Medicine 354*, 1157–1165.

Jennings, B. (2000) A life greater than the sum of its sensations: ethics, dementia, and the quality of life. In S.M. Albert and R.G. Logsdon (eds), *Assessing Quality of Life in Alzheimer's Disease.* New York, NY: Springer Publishing Co.

Jolley, D.J. and Benbow, S.M. (2000) Stigma and Alzheimer's disease: causes, consequences and a constructive approach. *International Journal of Clinical Practice 54*, (2), 117–119.

Joseph, J.A., Denisova, N.A., Bielinski, D., Fisher, D.R. and Shukitt-Hale, B. (2000) Oxidative stress protection and vulnerability in aging: putative nutritional implications for intervention. *Mechanisms of Aging and Development 116*, (2–3), 141–153.

Kasl-Godley, J. and Gatz, M. (2000) Psychosocial interventions for individuals with dementia: an integration of theory, therapy, and a clinical understanding of dementia. *Clinical Psychology Review 20*, (6), 755–782.

Khalsa, D.S. (1998) Integrated medicine and the prevention and reversal of memory loss. *Alternative Therapies in Health and Medicine 4*, (6), 38–43.

Kinney, J.M., Kart, C.S., Murdoch, L.D. and Conley, C.J. (2004) Striving to provide safety assistance for families of elders: the SAFE House project. *Dementia 3*, 351–370.

Klein, P.J. and Adams, W.D. (2004) Comprehensive therapeutic benefits of Taiji. A critical review. *American Journal of Physical Medicine and Rehabilitation 83*, (9), 735–745.

Knopman, D.S., Boeve, B.F. and Peterson, R.C. (2003) Essentials of the proper diagnoses of mild cognitive impairment, dementia, and major subtypes of dementia. *Mayo Clinical Proceedings 78*, 1290–1380.

LaBarge, E. and Trtanj, F. (1995) A support group for people in the early stages of dementia of the Alzheimer's type. *Journal of Applied Gerontology 14*, (3), 289–301.

Labarge, E., Von Dras, D. and Wingbermuehle, C. (1998) An analysis of themes and feelings from a support group for people with Alzheimer's disease. *Psychotherapy 35*, (4), 537–544.

Lekeu, F., Vojtasik, V., Van der Linden, M. and Salmon, E. (2002) Training early Alzheimer patients to use a mobile phone. *Acta Neurology of Belgium 102*, 114–121.

Luchsinger J.A. and Mayeux, R. (2004) Dietary factors and Alzheimer's disease. *The Lancet 3*, 579–587.

Lyman, K.A. (1989) Bringing the social back in: a critique of the biomedicalization of dementia. *The Gerontologist 29*, 597–606.

McCurry, S.M., Gibbon, L.E., Logsdon, R.G., Vitiello, M.V. and Teri, L. (2005) Nighttime insomnia treatment and education for Alzheimer's disease: a randomized, controlled trial. *Journal of the American Geriatrics Society 53*, (5), 793–802.

McIntosh, I.B., Swanson, V., Power, K.G. and Rae, C.A.L. (1999) General practitioners' and nurses' perceived roles, attitudes, and stressors in the management of people with dementia. *Health Bulletin 57*, (1), 35–40.

Mahendra, N. and Arkin, S. M. (2004). Exercise and volunteer work: contexts for AD language and memory interventions. *Seminars in Speech and Language 25*, (2), 151–167.

Mahendra, N., and Arkin, S. (2003). Effects of four years of exercise, language, and social interventions on Alzheimer discourse. *Journal of Communication Disorders 36*, (5), 395–422.

Markowitz, F.E. (1998) The effects of stigma on the psychological well-being and life satisfaction of persons with mental illness. *Journal of Health and Social Behavior 39*, 335–347.

Morhardt, D. and Johnson, N. (1998, November) *Effects of Memory Loss Support Groups for Persons with Early Stage Dementia and Their Families*. Paper presented at the meeting of the Gerontological Society of America, Philadelphia.

Morhardt, D., Sherrell, K. and Gross, B. (2003) Reflections of an early stage memory loss support group for persons with Alzheimer's and their family members. *Alzheimer's Care Quarterly 4*, (3), 185–188.

Oriani, M., Moniz-Cook, E., Binetti, G., Zanieri, G. *et al.* (2003) An electronic memory aid to support prospective memory in patients in the early stages of Alzheimer's disease: a pilot study. *Aging and Mental Health 7*, (1), 22–27.

Orrell, M., Spector, A., Thorgrimsen, L. and Woods, B. (2005). A pilot study examining the effectiveness of maintenance cognitive stimulation therapy (MCST) for people with dementia. *International Journal of Geriatric Psychiatry 20*, (5), 446–451.

Palo-Bengtsson, L. and Ekman, S.L. (2002) Emotional response to social dancing and walks in persons with dementia. *American Journal of Alzheimer's Disease and Other Dementias 17*, (3), 149–153.

Palo-Bengtsson, L., Winblad, B. and Ekman, S.L. (1998) Social dancing: a way to support intellectual, emotional and motor functions in persons with dementia. *Journal of Psychiatric and Mental Health Nursing 5*, 545–554.

Power, Rev. J. (2006) Religious and spiritual care. *Nursing Older People 18*, (7), 24–27.

Pearce, A., Clare, L. and Pistrang, N. (2002) Managing sense of self: coping in the early stages of Alzheimer's disease. *Dementia 1*, (2), 173–192.

Perkinson, M.A., Berg-Weger, M.L., Carr, D.B., Meuser, T.M., Palmer, J.L., Buckler, V.D. *et al.* (2005) Driving and dementia of the Alzheimer type: beliefs and cessation strategies among stakeholders. *The Gerontologist 45*, 676–685.

Quayhagen, M.P. and Quayhagen, M. (1996) Discovering life quality in coping in dementia. *Western Journal of Nursing Research 18*, (2), 120–135.

Rebok, G.W., Keyl, P.M., Bylsma, F.W., Blaustein, M.J. and Tune, L. (1994) The effects of Alzheimer disease on driving-related abilities. *Alzheimer Disease and Associated Disorders 8*, 228–240.

Rentz, C.A. (2002) Memories in the Making ©: outcome-based evaluation of an art program for individuals with dementing illnesses. *American Journal of Alzheimer's Disease and Other Dementias 17*, (3), 175–181.

Roger, K.S. (2006) Understanding social changes in the experience of dementia. *Alzheimer's Care Quarterly 7*, (3), 185–193.

Sabat, S.R. (2002) Selfhood and Alzheimer's disease. In P.B. Harris (ed.), *The Person with Alzheimer's Disease: Pathways to Understanding the Experience*. Baltimore, MD: The Johns Hopkins Press.

Sanglier, I., Sarazin, M. and Zinetti, J. (2004) Tai Chi, body and cognitive rehabilitation of Alzheimer's and related diseases. *Soins 685*, 42–43.

Sattin, R.W. (1992) Falls among older persons: a public health perspective. *Annual Review of Public Health 13*, 489–508.

Schreiber, M., Schweizer, A., Lutz, K., Kalveram, K.L. and Jancke, L. (1999) Potential of an interactive computer-based training in the rehabilitation of dementia: an initial study. *Neuropsychological Rehabilitation 9*, 155–167.

Sezaki, S. and Bloomgarden, J. (2002) Home-based art therapy for older adults. *Journal of the American Art Therapy Association 17*, (4), 283–290.

Small, G.W., Rabins, P.W., Barry, P., Buckholz, N.A., DeKoslay, S.T., Ferns, S.H. *et al.* (1997). Diagnosis and treatment of Alzheimer disease and related disorders: Consensus statement of the American Association for Geriatric Psychiatry, the Alzheimer's Association, and the American Geriatrics Society. *Journal of the American Medical Association 278*, 1363–1371.

Stansell, J. (2002) Volunteerism: contributions by persons with Alzheimer's disease. In P.B. Harris (ed.), *The Person with Alzheimer's Disease: Pathways to Understanding the Experience*. Baltimore, MD: The Johns Hopkins Press.

Teri, L., Gibbons, L.E., McCurry, S.M., Logsdon, R.G. *et al.* (2003) Exercise plus behavioral management in patients with Alzheimer disease. *Journal of the American Medical Association 290*, (15), 2015–2022.

Ting, D.Y. (2006) Certain hope. *Patient Education and Counseling 61*, 317–318.

Van Praag, H., Christie, B.R., Sejnowski, T.J. and Gage, F.H. (1999) Running enhances neurogenesis, learning, and long-term potentiation in mice. *Proceedings of the National Academy of Sciences USA 96*, (23), 13,427–13,431.

Vellone, E., Rega, M.L., Galletti, C. and Cohen, M.Z. (2006) Hope and related variables in Italian cancer patients. *Cancer Nursing 29*, (5), 356–364.

Vitiello, M.V., Prinz, P.N., Williams, D.E., Frommlet, M.S. and Ries, R.K. (1990) Sleep disturbances in patients with mild-stage Alzheimer's disease. *Journal of Gerontology 45*, (4), M131–M138.

Weinstein, L., and Xie, X. (1995) Purpose in life, boredom, and volunteerism in a group of elderly retirees. *Psychological Reports 76*, 482.

Woods, C.L., Moniz-Cook, E.D., Orrell, M. and Spector, A. (2006) Cognitive rehabilitation and cognitive training for early-stage Alzheimer's disease and vascular dementia (Review). *The Cochrane Collaboration*. Wiley Publishers.

Wright, L. (1993) *Alzheimer's Disease and Marriage*. Newbury Park, CA: Sage Publications.

Wu, G. (2002) Evaluation of the effectiveness of Tai Chi for improving balance and preventing falls in the older population—a review. *Journal of the American Geriatrics Society 50*, (4), 746–754.

Zarit, S.H., Femia, E.D., Watson, J., Rice-Oeschger, L. and Kakos, B. (2004) Memory club: a group intervention for people with early-stage dementia and their care partners. *The Gerontologist 44*, (2), 262–269.

Zeltzer, B.B., Stanley, S.S., Melo, L. and LaPorte, K.M. (2003) Art therapies promote wellness in elders. *Behavioral Healthcare Tomorrow* April, 7–12.

Yale, R. (1998, November). *Support Groups for Newly Diagnosed, Early Stage Alzheimer's Patients: How Patients Manage their Concerns*. Paper presented at the meeting of the Gerontological Society of America Annual Research Conference, Philadelphia, PA.

Index